SIRTFOOD DIET

A COMPREHENSIVE GUIDE TO LOSING WEIGHT, BURNING FAT, AND GETTING LEAN BY ACTIVATING THE POWER OF SIRTUINS AND THE SKINNY GENE. STAY HEALTHY, FIT, AND YOUNG BY EATING WHAT YOU LOVE!

ADELE WHITE

Text Copyright © [Adele White]

Legal & Disclaimer

The information contained in this book and its contents is not designed to replace or take the place of any form of medical or professional advice; and is not meant to replace the need for independent medical, financial, legal or other professional advice or services, as may be required. The content and information in this book has been provided for educational and entertainment purposes only.

The content and information contained in this book has been compiled from sources deemed reliable, and it is accurate to the best of the Author's knowledge, information and belief. However, the Author cannot guarantee its accuracy and validity and cannot be held liable for any errors and/or omissions. Further, changes are periodically made to this book as and when needed. Where appropriate and/or necessary, you must consult a professional (including but not limited to your doctor, attorney, financial advisor or such other professional advisor) before using any of the suggested remedies, techniques, or information in this book.

Upon using the contents and information contained in this book, you agree to hold harmless the Author from and against any damages, costs, and expenses, including any legal fees potentially resulting from the application of any of the information provided by this book. This disclaimer applies to any loss, damages or injury caused by the use and application, whether directly or indirectly, of any advice or information presented, whether for breach of contract, tort, negligence, personal injury, criminal intent, or under any other cause of action.

You agree to accept all risks of using the information presented inside this book.

You agree that by continuing to read this book, where appropriate and/or necessary, you shall consult a professional (including but not limited to your doctor, attorney, or financial advisor or such other advisor as needed) before using any of the suggested remedies, techniques, or information in this book.

Table of Contents

Introduction

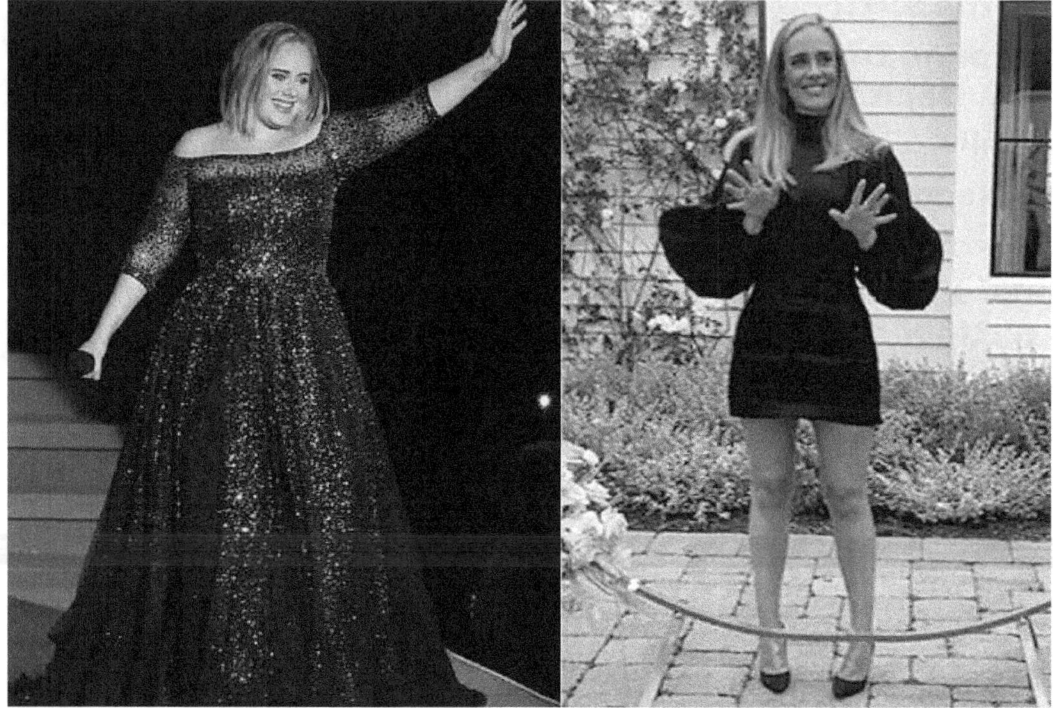

There is a wide variety of diets out there to choose from, and at the end of the day, it's all about finding what best for you. The Sirtfood diet, which eats plan stars like Adele and swears by Pippa Middleton, is one of the latest to grow in popularity. Let's walk over exactly what the Sirtfood diet is before you talk about trying it out for yourself.

The Sirtfood diet derives from the idea that certain proteins called Sirtuin or descriptively called "skinny genes" are activated by consuming certain items, and that they have the same effect as exercise or fasting by controlling the caloric consumption and eating foods containing a great deal of Sirtuin ("Sirtfood").

The Science Behind Sirtfood Diet

As such, we can consider every new diet through a prism of positive skepticism. The latest to generate news is the Sirtfood diet, which will assist with weight loss and other advantages such as "stimulating rejuvenation and cellular recovery" if we are to accept arguments at face value.

This sounds good—and Sirtuins are generally active in a broad range of cellular processes, including aging, growth, and circadian rhythm. The diet is often partially focused on limiting calories. The nutritionists behind this suggest the diet "influences the ability of the body to burn fat and enhance the metabolic system."

And what do we think about the diet? The answer from a scientific point of view is very little. In response to changes in energy levels, Sirtuin contributes to the regulation of fat and glucose metabolism. They can also play a role in improving the impact of calorie restrictions on aging. This may be via the effects of Sirtuin on aerobic (or mitochondrial) metabolism, decreasing species of reactive oxygen (free radicals), and increasing antioxidant enzymes.

Work also shows that transgenic mice with elevated SIRT6 rates live considerably longer than wild-type mice and that improvements in SIRT6 expression could be related to the aging of certain human skin cells. Also, slow metazoan (yeast) aging has been shown in SIRT2. It sounds amazing, and the diet has some positive feedback, but none of this is convincing empirical proof of the Sirtfood Diet having a comparable impact on actual people. Thinking that laboratory work on rodents, yeast, and human stem cells had some effect on real-world health results—

contaminated as they are by a plethora of confusing factors—will be a monumental over-extrapolation.

Weight Reduction Science

Doubtless for certain citizens, the diet would appear to fit. Yet empirical evidence of the results of every diet is still a separate thing. Of course, the optimal research to determine the feasibility of a weight loss program (or some other result, such as aging) will involve a reasonably broad survey—reflective of the demographic we're interested in—and random distribution to a treatment or control category. Outcomes will then be tracked over a reasonable period of time with tight control over confounding factors, such as certain activities that can impact value outcomes positively or adversely (smoking, example, or exercise).

Methods such as self-reporting and memory will restrict this study but will go some distance to explore the feasibility of this diet. Nevertheless, work of this type does not happen, and so we can be vigilant when analyzing fundamental science. After all, human cells in a tissue culture dish are likely to respond very differently to the cells of a living individual.

When we examine some of the basic arguments, more uncertainty is thrown on this diet. Losses of seven pounds in one week are unsustainable and are extremely unlikely to demonstrate body fat shifts. Dieters eat approximately 1000 kcal a day over the first three days— about 40-50 percent of what other people use. This would result in a rapid depletion of glycogen from the skeletal muscle and the liver (a processed source of carbohydrate).

But we also store around 2.7 grams of water for every gram of stored glycogen, and the water is high. But we do sacrifice corresponding oxygen with all the expended glycogen—and thus weight. Additionally, very stringent foods are very difficult to obey and result in elevated appetite-stimulating hormones, such as ghrelin. Hence, weight (glycogen and water) should return to usual if the temptation to feed is gaining.

In fact, it is challenging to adopt the empirical method to the study of diet. Often, placebo-controlled experiments of some degree of biological integrity are not feasible, and the clinical effects that we are all involved in carrying out for several years render study design difficult. In comparison, experiments of broad communities depend on remarkably simple and naïve forms of data collection, such as recall and self-reporting, which yield extremely inaccurate results. Health work has a tough job against environmental noise.

The Discovery and History of Sirtuin

In the 1970s, geneticist Dr. Amar Klara identified the first Sirtuin, dubbed SIR2, defining it as a gene that regulated yeast cells' capacity to fit. Years after, in the 1990s, researchers identified certain genes homologous—identical in function—to SIR2 in other species such as mice, fruit flies, and then called these SIR2 homologs Sirtuin. Every organism had a different number of Sirtuin. For example, yeast has five Sirtuin, one has bacteria, seven have mice, and seven have humans.

In 1991, alongside graduate students, Nick Austria and Brian Kennedy, Elysium co-founder, and MIT biologist Leonard Guarente performed experiments to grasp better how yeast agreed. By mistake, Austria decided to cultivate colonies of various yeast strains from samples that he had kept for months in his fridge, causing a hostile atmosphere for the strains. Just a few of these strains will grow here, but a pattern was identified by Guarente and his team: the longest-lived strains of yeast that survived the best in the fridge. This offered Guarente instructions so that he could concentrate exclusively on certain long-living yeast strains.

That led to SIR2 being identified as a gene that promoted yeast longevity. There is also no current evidence that this work can be extrapolated to people, and more research on the effects of SIR2 on people is needed. The Guarente lab thus observed that eliminating SIR2 significantly reduced yeast life, while, most notably, raising the number of copies of the SIR2 gene from one to two expanded the yeast life period. But, naturally, what activated SIR2 had yet to be found.

It is here where the acetyl classes come into action. Initially, it was thought that SIR2 could be a deacetylation enzyme—meaning it removed those acetyl groups—from other molecules, but nobody knew if this was true, because all try to show this operation was negative in the test tube. In Guarente's own words: "SIR2 does nothing without the NAD+." That was the crucial discovery of Sirtuin biology on the arc.

Benefits of Sirtfood Diet

While it is still fully researched and explored, the evidence currently points out that there is a wide range of benefits to the use of sirtuin activation. You can see all sorts of dietary benefits to this particular regimen that will overall make you a much healthier person. Currently, it is believed that you can find all sorts of real, compelling benefits if you made use of this diet on the regular, and that is promising. Let's go over some of the most common benefits now, and keep in mind that as of now, there is evidence to suggest this, but more research will need to be done over time.

You Will Lose Weight

The most obvious of the benefits is that you will lose weight on this diet. Whether you are exercising or not, there is no way that you would not lose weight when you follow the diet to a T. This diet will have you restrict your calories enough that anyone would lose weight. The average person uses around 2000 calories per day, and this diet will work to have you cut that in half; you will be providing yourself with just 1000 or 1500 calories based on the phase that you are in.

A calorie deficit causes weight loss—it is as simple as that. When you restrict your calories, but you keep your metabolism up, you will find that you will naturally lose weight. This is normal. However, usually, that weight loss is a mix of fat and muscle. As you lose weight and muscle, you would then naturally see your metabolism slow as well. Of course, this means that over time, your weight loss plan is not nearly as effective as it was supposed to be, and as a direct result, you will have to cut calories further to keep that deficit between consumed calories and the calories that your body naturally burns. This means that weight loss eventually slows, or even plateaus if all you do is make use of a weight-loss regimen through cutting calories. You will lose muscle if you are not careful with the weight loss regimen, and that will work against you.

However, thanks to the fact that you do not lose muscle mass during the Sirtfood Diet, you do not have to worry about this problem; you simply continue to lose weight because you are able to maintain your metabolism at levels that will be conducive to you continuing to lose that weight.

Your Appetite Will Slow

Although your first few days you may find that you are ravenous as your body adjusts to its new normal, over time, you should find that your diet will begin to slow down. Your body will adjust to the restrictions in calories, and you will be okay with the lower calorie days, especially because the food that you will be eating will include nutrient-dense food that will help your body feel like it is more satisfied. Lentils and buckwheat are very dense foods that are featured heavily in this diet, and you are able to add healthy fats, such as olive oil, to your diet so that you can feel truly satisfied, knowing that ultimately, you have given yourself enough to keep your body going. You will find that you will be able to tolerate the lower amounts of food, and that is a huge plus.

Pros & Cons of Sirtfood Diet

The greatest pro is that this lifestyle strongly promotes red wine, dark chocolate, and coffee, and it's not something you always read!

The compounds which make up our favorite treats are rich in activators of Sirtuin. Though drinking a kale smoothie, of course, followed by a whole bar of Green and Blacks will not see you dropping the pounds. Everything in balance. Aiden and Glen claim attendees never feel hunger – which suggests it's perfect for someone who can't get through a regular cleanse day without feeling like they're going to die because they do not have a Big Mac right away.

The Plan's first week is pretty intense. Days one and three are the most concentrated with a maximum calorie consumption of 1000—a mixture of three drinks and one dinner. Day's four to seven are marginally lenient with an average calorie of 1,500 calories a day. Few of the Pros & Cons are as below:

Pros:

- The 'sort foods' are meant to activate your body's Sirtuin, which is a form of protein that helps prevent your cells from dying and contracting diseases and controls your metabolism.

- It is based on a survey carried out by 40 gym-goers who each shed on average 7 lb. in a week without losing muscle mass.

- You should frequently have small doses of dark chocolate and champagne, without feeling guilty!

- This is built to be long-term and to maintain you alive for life and to delay the aging cycle.

Cons:

- For the first week, this is a calorie limit that would undoubtedly cause some people to lose weight regardless of what food is consumed. This means that the subjects could be gaining weight owing to the calorie limitation itself. You only eat 1,000 calories a day over the first three days, while the four days are 1,500 calories a day.

- Restricting your calorie consumption dramatically can be harmful when your body is accustomed to it and can render you feel lethargic.

- There is not enough proof that its claims, particularly the enhancement of your metabolism, carry through. 40-person research is not big enough to suggest it would necessarily act as a safe way to lose weight.

- Just items including 'sort juices,' green tea, rocket, soy, and walnuts may be on the sort food list.

- Less focus is put on bringing a range of foods into your diet so you can look and sound fantastic. Feeding a rainbow of fruit and veg every day, for example, means you bring a range of vitamins and minerals into your diet.

The Sirtfood Diet is full of nutritious foods, but eating habits are not pleasant. This hypothesis and safety arguments are, not to mention, found on large extrapolations from sparse empirical facts. Although it isn't a terrible thing to attach any products to the diet and might even provide certain health benefits, the diet itself seems like yet another fad. Save the money and skip healthy, long-term nutritional changes instead.

Chapter 1. What Are Sirtuins?

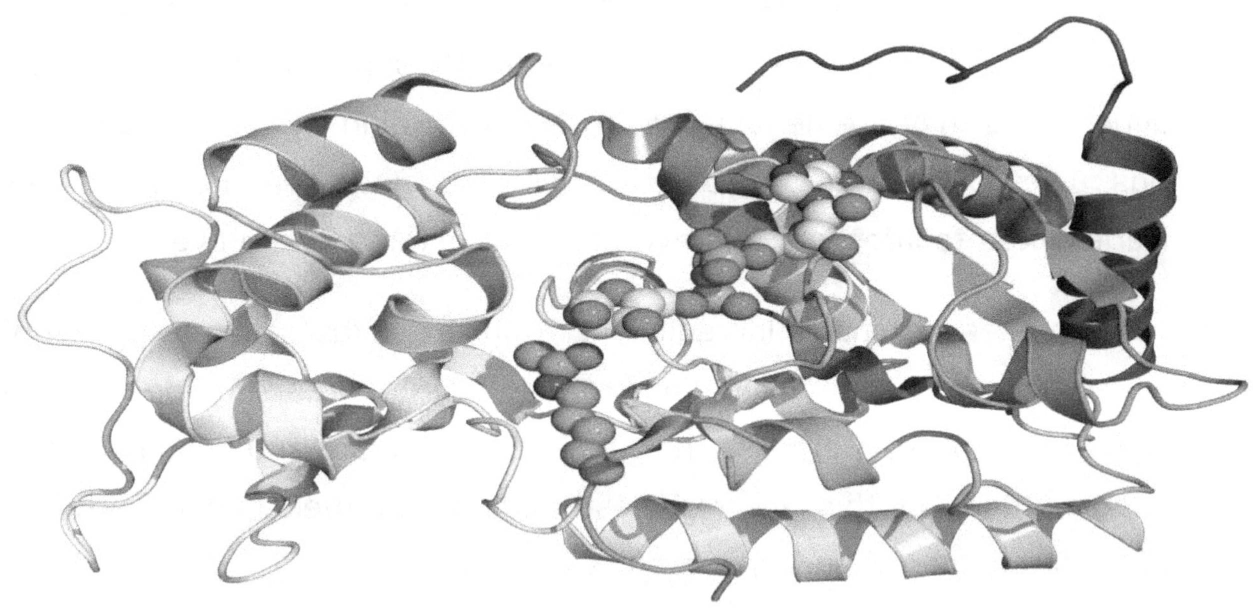

Sirtuins are a kind of protein, which shield the cells in our bodies from getting aggravated through the sickness. However, it has recently demonstrated they can help manage your digestion, the assists in an increment of muscle and consume fat—thus tagging along by its new name 'superfood'.

Sirtuins are a class of proteins that have either mono-ADP-ribosyltransferase or deacetylase action, including deacetylase, desuccinylase, deadenylase, demyristoylase and depalmitoylase movement. The name Sir2 originates from the yeast quality 'quiet mating-type data guideline 2,' the quality liable for cell guideline in yeast.

Sirtuins: "Skinny Gene" Activator?

Individuals have consistently been entranced with questions about how we can live more and more advantageous lives. Indeed, mainstream researchers have a similar interest with a group of qualities called sirtuins. All of us houses sirtuins—frequently alluded to as our thin qualities—and they are genuinely entrancing, holding the ability to decide things like our capacity to consume fat and remain slim, our powerlessness to infection, and even to what extent we can live.

So what makes sirtuins so incredible? Sirtuins are extraordinary in view of their capacity to change our phones to a sort of endurance mode—setting off a fantastic reusing process that gets out cell waste and consumes fat. The advantages of this are truly astounding: fat melts away, and we become fitter, more slender, and more beneficial.

How Can We Utilize Sirtuins?

This brings up the issue: what would we be able to do to actuate sirtuins and receive these astonishing rewards? It is notable that both fasting and exercise enact sirtuins. Be that as it may, oh dear, both interest an unfaltering promise to either food limitation or requesting exercise systems. Reducing calories leaves us feeling exhausted, hungry, and unequivocally irritable, and in the more drawn out term can prompt muscle misfortune and stale digestion. With respect to work out, the sum should have been compelling for weight reduction requires a LOT of exertion. Both can be difficult to achieve.

In 2013, the consequences of one of the most esteemed nourishing examinations at any point completed were distributed. The reason for the evaluation, called PREDIMED, was flawlessly straightforward: It considered the contrast between a Mediterranean-style diet enhanced with either extra-virgin olive oil or nuts and a progressively traditional present-day diet. Results indicated that following five years, coronary illness and diabetes were cut by an extraordinary 30 per cent, alongside significant decreases in the danger of heftiness in the Mediterranean eating regimen gathering. This wasn't unexpected, yet when the examination was explored in more exceptional detail, it was found there was no distinction in calorie, fat, or sugar consumption between the two gatherings. How would you clarify that?

Not every food is made equivalent. Research currently shows that plants contain regular mixes called polyphenols that have enormous advantages for our wellbeing. What's more, when analysts dissected PREDIMED researched polyphenol utilization among the members, the outcomes faltered. Over only the five-year time frame, the individuals who expended the most significant levels of polyphenols had 37 per cent fewer passing, contrasted with the individuals who ate the least.

Be that as it may, not all polyphenols are equivalent. Information out of Harvard University from more than 124,000 people indicated that certain lone polyphenols were useful for weight control. Thus, an investigation of around 3,000 twins found that a higher admission of just certain polyphenols was connected with less muscle versus fat and a more beneficial circulation of fat in the body. Polyphenols are without a doubt a shelter for remaining thin and robust, yet in the event that not all polyphenols are equivalent, at that point, which is the best? Would it be able to be those that examination has indicated have the capacity to turn on our sirtuin qualities? Exactly the same ones actuated by fasting and exercise?

The pharmaceutical business has rushed to abuse these sirtuin-enacting supplements, contributing many millions to change over them into panacea drugs. For instance, mainstream diabetes tranquillizes metformin originates from a plant and actuates our sirtuin qualities. In any case, as of recently, they have been to a great extent ignored by the universe of nourishment, to the disservice of our wellbeing and our waistlines.

What Nutrients Activate Sirtuins?

We put all the nourishments with the most significant levels of sirtuin-actuating polyphenols together into a different eating regimen with our advantage aroused. This incorporates extra-virgin olive oil and pecans, the particular considerations in PREDIMED, just as arugula, red onions, strawberries, red wine, dim chocolate, green tea, and espresso, among numerous others. At the point when we pilot tried it, the outcomes were shocking. Members shed pounds while either keeping up or, in any event, expanding their bulk. The best part is that individuals detailed inclination extraordinary—overflowing with vitality, resting better, and with remarkable upgrades in their skin.

Thus the Sirtfood Diet was conceived, a progressive better approach to enact sirtuins by eating heavenly nourishments. An eating routine that doesn't include calorie forgetting about, removing carbs, or eating low fat. An eating routine of consideration in which you receive the rewards from eating the nourishments your adoration. The Sirtfood Diet is shaking things up of right dieting guidance and what it truly intends to look and feel incredible. And all from eating our preferred nourishments!

Fasting Versus Calorie Limitation

Supplement hardship or supplement pressure likely incorporates numerous dietary limitation types, including calorie/dietary limitation, time confined eating regimen (tRD), discontinuous fasting, and fasting. Calorie/dietary limitation depicts the decrease in calorie consumption by generally 20–30%. A period confined eating regimen portrays one supper for each day with typical day by day calorie admission. Intermittent fasting is substituting long periods of standard eating routine and fasting, while unadulterated fasting is finished food starvation for a few backs to back days. In spite of the fact that calorie/dietary limitation has been appeared to influence life expectancy emphatically and disease treatment in research facility settings, interpretation of clinical investigations has been restricted for a few reasons.

In the first place, interminable calorie/dietary limitation has been appeared just to defer the movement of tumor development, and this postpone will happen only for a subset of malignancies. Likewise, the weight reduction and debilitating of the invulnerable framework made by calorie/dietary limitation make it hard for disease patients to experience chemotherapy. On the other hand, a tRD and additional discontinuous fasting displayed comparative impacts contrasted with calorie/dietary limitation; however, they don't bring about weight reduction and can be increasingly mediocre in patients. The main burden for tRD, discontinuous fasting, and even calorie/dietary limitation is that they require an all-inclusive time before any insurance produces results that may confine the potential use in malignant growth treatment.

At long last, fasting quickly preceding chemotherapy treatment followed by the arrival to the healthy eating regimen doesn't cause weight reduction in the long haul while possibly upgrading the valuable impacts of chemotherapy. Nonetheless, is it convenient for a malignancy quiet experiencing delayed fasting? Albeit a few examinations have demonstrated that slow starvation is endured in patients with interminable ailments and proposed to be very much taken, it is mentally awkward for some patients. In light of these investigations, it is sensible to suggest that a tRD and additionally discontinuous fasting may accomplish comparative objectives contrasted with calorie/dietary limitation yet with fewer reactions and in that capacity, be increasingly valuable in clinical malignancy treatment, though drawn out fasting might be progressively successful for disease avoidance.

The gainful impacts of fasting have been exhibited for a long time, and all through the typical course of a living being's life, changes in accessible supplements are healthy, and times of starvation are normal. Versatile reactions have created over the life form's advancement to shield it from conceivably deadly threats during these times of famine from any of various potential natural conditions. Numerous past and late investigations have indicated that starvation-actuated pressure opposition is clear and rationed in a wide range of animal types. In both yeast and Escherichia coli, glucose starvation expands assurance against oxidative pressure and, in yeast alone, even a critical increment in life span. Worms and flies appeared to profit by the equivalent expanded obstruction against oxidative worry after starvation attributable to the redirection of vitality from cell development to insurance. Various investigations additionally show that fasting ensures the rodent cerebrum, mouse kidney and liver, and human liver from ischemia injury.

Also, starvation or a 10–30% reduction in calorie consumption builds life expectancy up to half and forestalls carcinogenesis in unconstrained, synthetic, or radiation-instigated tumorigenesis in a few mammalian test models. Progressively significant, late investigations further recommend that fasting can crosstalk with sirtuins, a life span quality family, which have been proposed to be essential in maturing and carcinogenesis.

Correlation with Inflammation/Insulin Resistance/Metabolism

When you restrict calories, you essentially tell your body that food is not available to it. You have a normal metabolism that is meant to tell you when to eat to make sure that you constantly have energy. Think of hunger like that little gas light coming on in your car—it is there to remind you that you are running low on stored gas and that filling it up soon would probably be a good idea. Your hunger is there to keep you topped off essentially—it does not want you to drop below a certain level. However, when you restrict your calories, you do not provide that extra food. This means that your body has to shift gears—it can no longer count on being topped off to provide the needed energy levels, and the deficit is created.

When that happens, the body has a great backup mechanism that your car does not. Your body has stores of fat that can be broken down when there is a deficit in calories. When your body cannot get what it requires, it can instead work to get those calories elsewhere; it can provide itself with energy by breaking down that fat. Does that sound familiar? It is quite like the function of the sirtuins! Essentially, due to the threat to homeostasis in the body, the sirtuins activate and inhibit insulin while encouraging the oxidation of the fat in the body.

Usually, during calorie restriction, there are also other side effects, such as losing muscle, but that will be able to be protected against in other ways. During mild to moderate calorie restriction, weight loss is normal and expected without too many other issues. One of the more common ways of creating a deficit in calories is through the use of exercising while also restricting calories.

Chapter 2. How to Change Bad Eating Habits

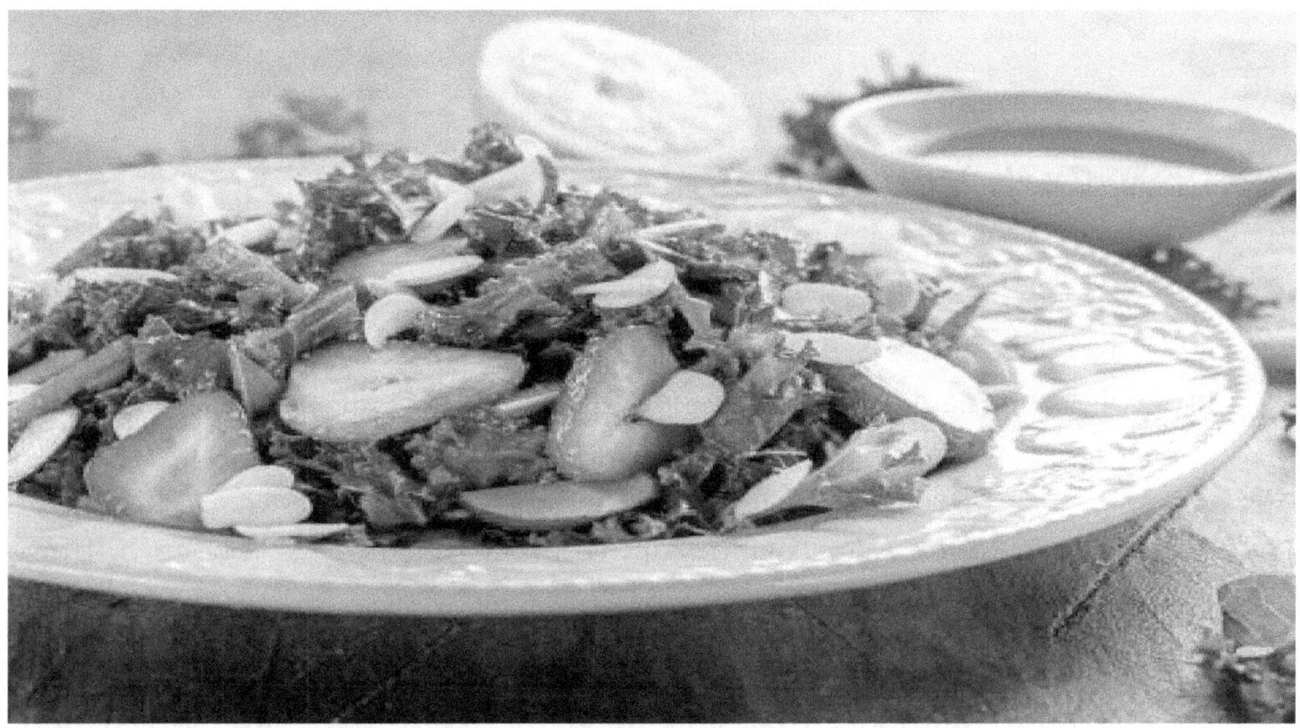

I've had people complain about the difficulty of switching their grocery list to one that's sirtfoods diet-friendly. The fact is that food is expensive—and most of the food you have in your fridge is probably packed full of carbohydrates. This is why if you're committing to a sirtfoods diet, you need to do a clean sweep. That's right—everything that's packed with carbohydrates should be identified and set aside to make sure you're not eating more than you should.

Seafood

Seafood means fish like sardines, mackerel, and wild salmon. It's also a good idea to add some shrimp, tuna, mussels, and crab into your diet.

This is going to be a tad expensive, but worth it in the long run. What's the common denominator in all these food items? The secret is omega-3 fatty acids, which are credited for lots of health benefits. You want to add food rich in omega-3 fatty acids to your diet.

Low-Carb Vegetables

The Vegetable Choices should be limited to those with low carbohydrate counts. Pack up your cart with items like spinach, eggplant, arugula, broccoli, and cauliflower. You can also put in bell peppers, cabbage, celery, kale, Brussels sprouts, mushrooms, zucchini, and fennel.

So what's in them? Well, aside from the fact that they're low-carb, these vegetables also contain loads of fiber, which makes digestion easier. Of course, there's also the presence of vitamins, minerals, antioxidants, and various other nutrients that you need for day-to-day life. Which ones should you avoid? Steer clear of the starch-packed vegetables like carrots, turnips, and beets. As a rule, you go for the plants that are green and leafy.

Fruits Low in Sugar

During an episode of sugar-craving, it's usually a good idea to pick low-sugar fruit items. Believe it or not, there are lots of those in the market! Just make sure to stock up on any of these: avocado, blackberries, raspberries, strawberries, blueberries, lime, lemon, and coconut. Also, note that tomatoes are fruits too, so feel free to make side dishes or dips with loads of vegetables! Keep in mind that these fruits should be eaten fresh and not out of a can. However, if you do eat them raw off the box, take a good look at the nutritional information at the back of the packaging. Avocadoes are particularly popular for those practicing the Sirtfood Diet because they contain LOTS of the right kind of fat.

Meat and Eggs

While some diets will tell you to skip the meat, the Sirtfood Diet encourages its consumption. Chicken is packed with protein that will feed your muscles and give you a consistent energy source throughout the day. It's a slow but sure burn when you eat protein as opposed to carbohydrates, which are burned faster and therefore stored faster if you don't use them immediately.

But what kind of meat should you be eating? There's chicken, beef, pork, venison, turkey, and lamb. Keep in mind that quality plays a huge role here—you should be eating grass-fed organic beef or organic poultry if you want to make the most out of this food variety. The nuclear option lets you limit the possibility of ingesting toxins in your body due to these products' production process. Plus, the preservation process also means added salt or sugar in the meat, which can throw off the whole diet.

Nuts and Seeds

Nuts and seeds you should add to your cart include chia seeds, brazil nuts, macadamia nuts, flaxseed, walnuts, hemp seeds, pecans, sesame seeds, almonds, hazelnut, and pumpkin seeds. They also contain lots of protein and very little sugar, so they're great if you have the munchies.

They're the ideal snack because they're quick, easy, and will keep you full. They're high in calories, though, which is why lots of people steer clear of them. As I mentioned earlier, though—the Sirtfoods Diet has nothing to do with calories and everything to do with the nutrient you're eating. So don't pay too much attention to the calorie count and just remember that they're a good source of fats and protein.

Dairy Products

Some people in their 50 already have a hard time processing dairy products, but for those who don't, you can happily add many of these to your diet. Make sure to consume sufficient amounts of cheese, plain Greek yogurt, cream butter, and cottage cheese. These dairy products are packed with calcium, protein, and a healthy kind of fat.

Coffee and Tea

The good news is that you don't have to skip coffee if you're going on a Sirtfoods Diet. The bad news is that you can't go to Starbucks anymore and order their blended coffee choices. Instead, beverages would be limited to unsweetened tea or unsweetened coffee to keep sugar consumption low—option for organic coffee and tea products to make the most out of these powerful antioxidants.

Dark Chocolate

Yes—chocolate is still on the menu, but it is limited to just dark chocolate. Technically, this means eating chocolate that is 70 percent cacao, which would make the taste a bit bitter.

Chapter 3. The Importance of Mindset for Reaching Your Target in Weight Loss

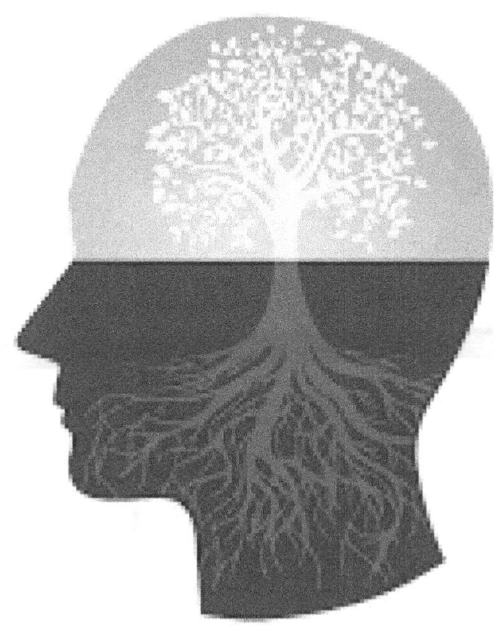

All diets work. All. Or, at least, the main ones. But not all dieters manage to lose weight.

This concept can be foreign to all fields of our life; for example, many people graduate with high marks, but few manage to get the job they dream of. Many people play basketball, but very few come to play in the NBA.

Why do some succeed and others fail? What more do they have to those who fail?

And, returning to the world of diets, why is losing weight so difficult?

The answer is The Mindset!

To be able to talk about it and to be able to exploit it, you must first define what the mindset is. With this expression, we want to refer, in general, to all that set of conditionings and beliefs that our mind has assimilated during life. This habitual mental attitude characterizes our ways of reacting and acting in certain circumstances. In a sense, we can define the mindset as our usual behavior in the face of situations that arise.

For example, if a subject is convinced that he cannot speak publicly, he will probably tend to avoid the occasions when it is necessary to show his skills in front of others. This determines a general insecurity, which if not addressed, will take root more and more deeply in his mind, causing him to give up and surrender for fear of making mistakes.

This is precisely one of the reasons why I find it essential to know yourself. Knowing what your limits are, your fears, your difficulties, and being able to admit them is an important step towards the possibility of overcoming your limits. Although they are often imaginary limits that we place ourselves when, in reality, our fears speak and make us believe that there are obstacles that cannot be overcome.

We assume that nothing presents such an insurmountable problem; sometimes, what is needed is to have the right weapons to deal with it and a little help to take the field and fight. We said that the mindset is a mental setting that has taken root in each of us year after year. So how is it possible to change what seems sedimented in us so deeply? The most appropriate answer to this question is that after having cleared what the mindset is, what there is to do is put it into practice.

Practicing is the best way to fix theoretical concepts concretely and start implementing good intentions. In short, the theory is necessary for knowledge purposes, but if it is not fixed by practice, it risks remaining at an end in itself. So, I invite you to translate your intentions into real and useful activities.

Obviously, it will be fundamental, first of all, to acquire a new mindset, changing it, and trying to introduce positive concepts into your mind that can be useful both in personal and professional life. After realizing what the mindset is, it is time to move on to implementation.

This step may not be so easy and immediate, and, above all, it may also happen that you do not immediately put the correct strategy into practice. This depends on the fact that there are rare times when it is possible to act already in the right and effective way. Different tactics correspond to each activity and situation.

This means that the transition to practice requires adjustments along the way. There is no definitive or right mindset in absolute and in all situations, but you will have to model your ad hoc strategies for every occasion. The mindset is not a point of arrival but a process in progress, a continuous evolution of the personal way of approaching things.

Mindset for a Successful Diet

Once we have explained what the mindset is and how it influences our way of thinking, we can explain the part that interests us most: how to use it to carry out a successful diet.

Let's start by saying that food, from a psychological point of view, represents a fundamental need for a human being: pleasure.

Now, if food is related to pleasure, and if pleasure is a fundamental emotion (even one of the 4 fundamental for our survival—the others are fear, anger, and pain), in your opinion, we can take the idea of depriving us of food?

Fast Until Explodes

What typically happens in all diets is this: follow them for "n" days and then stop. At best. In the worst, you follow them for n days and then explode in a binge that makes you recover all the pounds lost with interest.

Think about something you like.

"Food?"

No, no, to anything else. Now, imagine depriving yourself of it for a while: how would you feel? How much would you miss? How much would you like it? How long would it be in your thoughts? And in your feelings? Are you hypnotizing yourself? No? Does nothing, so the concept is clear, right? Depriving ourselves of something we like makes us want even more.

This criterion is practically universal, and you find it in any situation: from courtship (where one of the two "subtracts" the other to be sought even more), up to marketing (where the things we like are put on a "limited offer" So that we can buy them immediately—in reality, this is also done with those we don't like, and we often find ourselves buying things that we don't really need).

In short, the more you deprive yourself of it, the more you desire it.

The Pleasant Diet

Dieting cannot be pleasant, make a reason for it. I mean: how pleasant can deprivation of pleasure be? Because then, mathematical law, all the best (and therefore pleasant) foods are those that are excluded from diets.

This reasoning is perhaps not fully valid with the Sirtfood Diet because many good foods can be eaten since they are superfoods. However, something can be done. First of all, a pleasant diet is such if there is a pleasure on the table. Eating is a perfect metaphor for sex here. Now, if you are a man, forget what I am about to say; you cannot understand. If, instead, you are a woman, answer this question: what are the pleasant moments of sex? I am pretty sure that you will not think exclusively (and perhaps not even first) about orgasm: you will think of a series of before, during, or after that make that experience really pleasant.

The feeling of caresses, the lips that touch the neck, even the slight pain of the teeth tightening on the skin. And again, the freshness of the sheets at the end of everything, or even before the choice of underwear to wear (dear man, I reveal a reality known to every woman: if when you undress for the first time she wears an intimate outfit, you are not who seduced her, it was she who had already decided to take you to bed), the background music, the heart that beats as you are entering the room... In short, pleasure is also in all this, not only in the blatant moments.

Likewise, eating must be a pleasure. If you do a diet, you should make sure that the whole outline is kept to make the moment as pleasant as possible. For example, it is usually more beautiful to eat with a minimum setting than to do it with a plastic plate or a sandwich wrapped in paper (and, if you eat outside, you can find a bench, a corner of greenery, or any other pleasant space); better to do it by listening to some music or in the pleasant sound of silence, than with the TV on or, worse, continuing to work; you should taste the food, don't just pass it from the mouth to the stomach.

And so on... If, on the contrary, you throw down the bitter (and poor) bite to finish what you consider torture as soon as possible, you are making it worse than it is. And you'll soon end up bursting.

Give in to Temptations

As said, then, the moment you deprive yourself of something pleasant, this becomes even more desired. So, what's the solution? That's right: give it up. Oscar Wilde said: "I can resist everything except temptations." But if I give it to myself, it will no longer be a temptation.

What does it mean?

It means that there should be spaces in your diet to give up, from time to time, to the thing you give up. An afternoon chocolate, a plate of pasta every now and then, a less restrictive Sunday... Without exaggerating, of course, but ensuring that the food denied is not permanently denied, otherwise it will be worse.

I know it seems paradoxical (and indeed it is), because I'm telling you to eat (every now and then, in a thoughtful way) just what you shouldn't be eating. But, tell me, did your tactic work this far?

The best way to resist a temptation is to indulge in special spaces just what we are taking away, in order to make the temptation less strong and to give us pleasure in small doses, which allow our diet to function properly. Eat to believe.

Chapter 4. Who Can Do the Sirtfood Diet and Who Cannot Do It

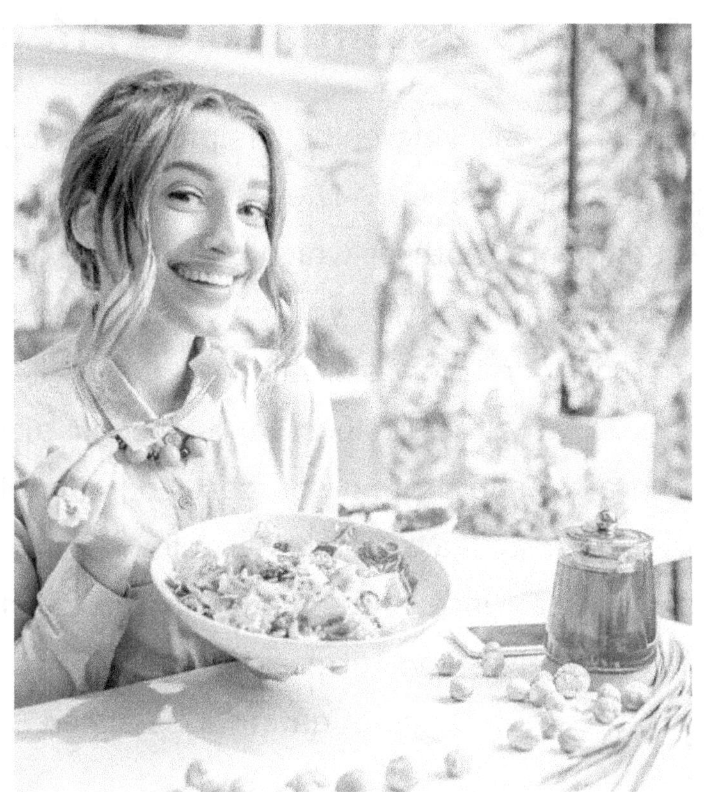

Who Should Try Sirtfood Diet?

The SirtFood diet is suitable for Individuals who:

- Are overweight or obese

- Want to maintain his/her weight

- Needs to have a "detox" and flush away the toxins from the body

- Have failed to lose weight using different diet techniques

- Want not only to lose weight but also build muscle

- Want a healthier lifestyle and to achieve optimal health

Sirt Diet Safety and Potential Side Effects

Foods rich in sirtuins are also incredibly helpful superfoods that anyone could benefit from eating more of. They are high in anti-inflammatory properties and antioxidants, both of which can reduce the risk of disease and slow down cellular aging. But, if you only choose to eat foods on the Sirt food list that I provided you above, then you will not be eating a balanced diet. This is why the recipes in this book also include other fruits, vegetables, grains, and protein sources. You cannot live off of only a handful of ingredients, at least not healthfully. If you try to eat only sirtuin-rich foods, you may lose more health in the short-term, but you will only experience negative long-term side effects. This is why I, again and again, promote the importance of eating a balanced Sirtfood diet.

The first phase of the Sirt diet can be restrictive, as you are eating one thousand to fifteen hundred calories a day. However, for this reason, the first phase only lasts a week and is healthy to do in the short-term. You wouldn't want to live an entire month eating that number of calories a day, but, for a week most, it is sufficient for most people. Regularly consult your family doctor before making big life changes that affect your health. Depending on your specific health, weight, and activity level, you might need to make an adjustment to a diet plan to make it work for your individual needs. Your doctor is the one most qualified to determine if you need to make these given adjustments. For instance, if you work a manual labour job, your doctor might recommend increasing your calorie and protein intake to keep your energy levels up. Remember, if your doctor does have concerns due to your individual health, it doesn't mean you can't follow the Sirt diet, simply that you need to make their recommended adjustments to your plan.

Thankfully, the average healthy adult is unlikely to have any problems with the Sirt diet if they follow it in a balanced manner recommended. This means you shouldn't increase the duration of phase one to promote further weight loss. Remember, if you want to lose more weight, then only repeat phase one after completing phase two.

For a healthy adult, the most common side effects are fatigue, irritability, and light-headedness. This is usually due to calorie restriction and can occur whenever a person goes on a diet or changes their eating habits.

You should also know that this diet is not recommended for anyone with an eating disorder. This is because while the calorie restriction is healthy when followed according to plan, it only reinforces their negative relationship with food for a person who already has disordered eating. The result could be that if someone with an eating disorder attempts to follow this or any other diet calling for counting calories that their eating disorder will likely worsen. Of course, if you or someone you know has an eating disorder and still wants to benefit from sirtuin-rich foods, you can still enjoy the recipes in this book and incorporate the top Sirtfoods into your daily meal plan without cutting your calorie intake. You may not experience as much weight loss, but you have to prioritize your mental health and healing from disordered eating.

To sum it up, you should speak with your doctor before drastically changing your eating habits no matter what diet you are trying, and that includes the Sirt diet. However, if you are healthy and not pregnant, breastfeeding, or suffering from an eating disorder, it should be safe if you follow the diet as recommended. Even if you have a chronic illness or disease, it may be healthy, but only your doctor can say for sure, as each person's disease, condition, and treatment will vary.

Chapter 5. How to Build a Diet That Works

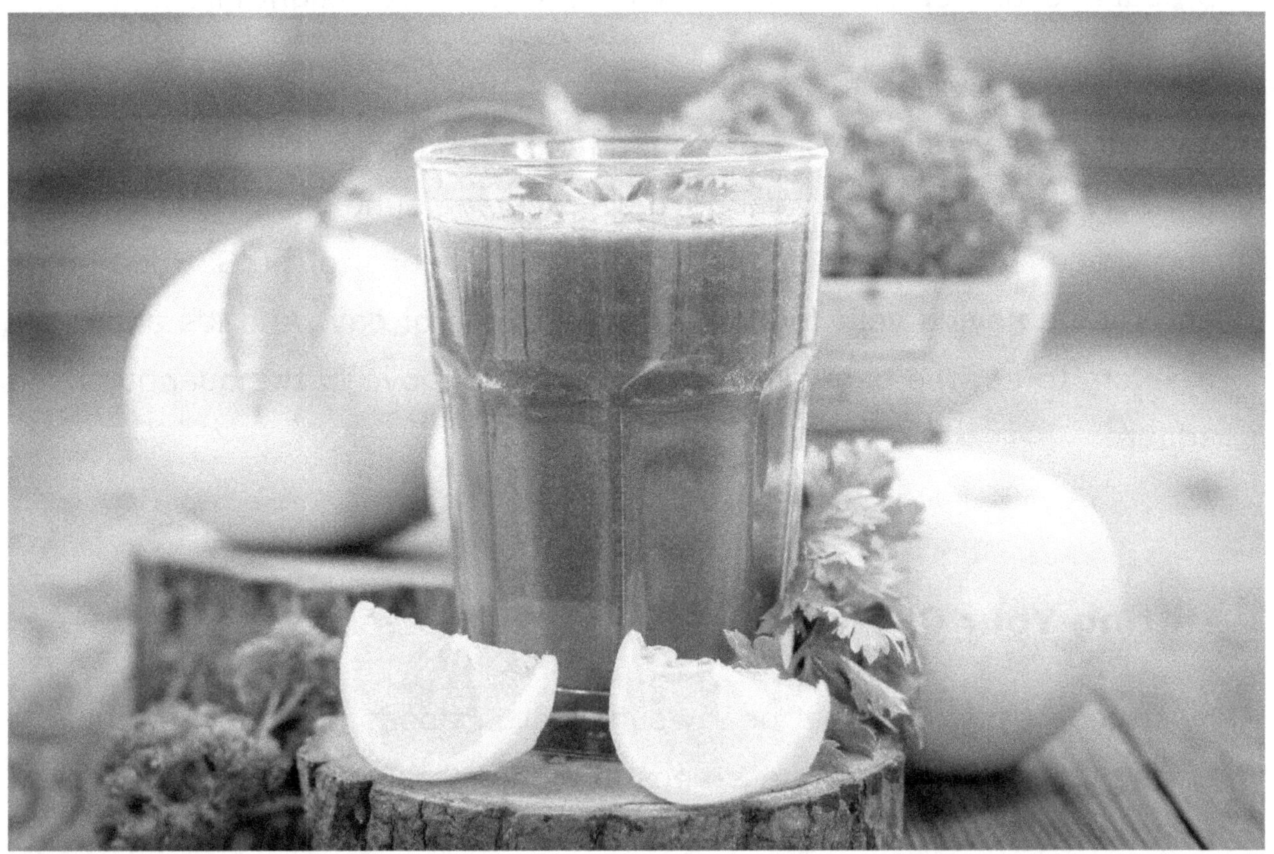

Tips to Build the Sirtfood Diet That Better Fits for You

We have done something very unique with the Sirtfood Diet. We took the most powerful Sirtfoods on the biosphere and knitted them into a brand-new healthy diet, the likes of which were not seen before. We picked the "best and brightest" from the healthful diets we have ever identified and built a world-beating recipe from them.

The great thing is you don't immediately have to follow an Okinawan's typical diet or eat like an Italian mamma. This on the Sirtfood Diet is not only utterly unfeasible, but also needless. Yes, one thing you may be taken by from the Sirtfoods list is their similarity. While you do not consume any of the items on the list at the moment, you are very much probably eating others. And why don't you just lose weight already?

When we analyze the various elements that the most chopping-edge nutrition science displays are required to build a workable diet, the issue is addressed. It is about eating the proper amount of Sirtfoods, range, and shape. It's about adding ample protein portions to the Sirtfood bowls and then enjoying your foods at the right time of day. And it's about the freedom to eat the genuinely savory foods you love in the quantities you admire.

Hitting Your Quota

Most people just don't eat nearly sufficient Sirtfoods right now to evoke a strong fat-burning and fitness-boosting influence. When the study looked at the US diet utilization of five main sirtuins-activating components (quercetin, luteolin, myricetin, kaempferol, and apigenin), human dietary intakes were found to be miserably thirteen milligrams a day. Conversely, the Japanese daily consumption was 5 times greater. Contrasting with our Sirtfood Diet experiment, every day, persons ate hundreds of milligrams of sirtuins-activating foods.

All we are speaking about is a true diet transformation in which we raise by as much as 50 times our daily consumption of sirtuins-activating components. Although that might seem overwhelming or unrealistic, it isn't necessarily. By taking all our highest level Sirtfoods and trying to put them together in a fully consistent manner with your stressful schedule, you can indeed efficiently and cheaply reach the level of consumption needed to gain all of the advantages.

The Power of Synergy

We think it is important to eat a vast array of these wonder nutrients as whole organic foods, where they coexist along with the dozens of other natural biologically active substances that work synergistically to increase our wellbeing. We think working with the natural world is best, instead of against. This is for this purpose that single nutrient supplementation does not display permanent effect time and time again, but the same component is represented in the form of an entire diet.

Take, for example, the basic component resveratrol, which activates sirtuin. This is partially consumed in supplementary form; but its bioavailability (how much more the individual can use) is at least 6 times higher in its normal food material of red wine. Refer to this the reality that red wine produces not only one but a complete variety of sirtuins-activating polyphenols that work with each other to offer positive effects, like myricetin, piceatannol, quercetin, and epicatechin. Perhaps we could direct our focus from the turmeric to curcumin. Curcumin is very well-established as the main sirtuins-activating ingredient in turmeric, but work reveals that this whole turmeric has stronger PPAR-ÿ action to combat fat burning and is much more capable of suppressing cancer and decreasing blood glucose levels than isolated curcumin. It's not hard to understand that trying to isolate a single nutrient in its full food process is still nowhere near as successful as eating it.

Yet, when we begin combining multiple Sirtfoods, what really makes a nutritional plan special is. For example, by trying to introduce it in quercetin-rich Sirtfoods, we enhance the impacts of resveratrol-containing foods a lot further. Not even just that, even in their conduct, they complement one another. All of those are fat blockers, but how either of them actually achieves that is complicated. Resveratrol is very effective in promoting the deterioration of mature fat cells, while quercetin is active in preventing new fat tissue from developing. In addition, they ingest food on both ends, leading to a high losing weight impact than consuming just large amounts of a single ingredient.

So, this is a method which we see again and again. Foods that are high in sirtuin enhancer apigenin boost the quercetin uptake from diet and increase its function. Quercetin, in effect, has been shown to be synergistic with epigallocatechin gallate (EGCG) activity. And EGCG's work with curcumin has been seen to be complementary. And so, it begins. Not only are whole individual products more effective than single ingredients, but we reach into yet another tapestry of beneficial effects that the natural world has blended—so deep, so pure, it's difficult to attempt to beat it.

Juicing and Food: Get the Best of Both Worlds

Sirtfood Diet is a portion of both juices and whole food products. There we are speaking about juices made directly from a juicer—blenders and milkshake makers (including the NutriBullet) do not work. For others, that may sound counterintuitive, based on the fact that the fiber is lost while juiced. Yet this is just what we need from leafy green vegetables.

Feed fiber includes what is termed non-extractable polyphenols (or NEPPs), which are polyphenols called sirtuin additives, which are bound to the fibrous portion of the food and only emitted by our helpful intestinal bacteria when decomposed. We don't even get the NEPPs by erasing the fiber and end up losing out on their righteousness. Crucially, though, the NEPP composition varies significantly based on the size of the plant. The NEPP material of a diet rich in fruits, cereals, and grains is meaningful and should be ingested whole (NEPPs provide over fifty percent of polyphenols in strawberries!). However, for leafy green vegetables, the essential compounds in the Sirtfood juice, they are much lesser even after having a bigger fiber content.

So, we get full value for our buck whenever it applies to leafy green vegetables by juicing them and eliminating the low-nutrient material, so we can use even increasing quantities and obtain an amazingly concentrated dose of sirtuins-activating polyphenols.

There is yet another benefit of cutting the fibers, too. Green leafy vegetables contain a form of fiber called non-soluble fiber, which has a gastrointestinal scrubbing action. However, when we consume so much of it, it will frustrate and hurt our digestive lining quite as if we over-scrub stuff. That ensures that for so many people, green leafy vegetables-packed smoothies can overwhelm fibred, possibly aggravating or even inducing IBS (irritable bowel syndrome) and hampering our nutrient uptake.

When it tends to come to digesting their goodness, having a few of your Sirtfoods in juice form can even have significant benefits. For instance, matcha green tea has been one of the additives we include in the green juice. When we eat the EGCG sirtuin activator present in high amounts of green tea in the form of drinks lacking milk, its ingestion is higher than sixty-five percent. We also found it important to remember that transitioning towards smoothies to green juices carried about significant rises in their quantities of other vital nutrients, including magnesium and folic acid, as we ran lab tests on our own customers.

The core issue of it all is that to get those sirtuin genetic factors ringing for massive weight loss and wellbeing, we have to establish an eating plan that incorporates for greatest advantage both juices and whole meals.

The Power of Protein

These are plants that bring the Sirt into the nutrition of Sirtfood, yet to get optimum value, Sirtfood foods will also have a high protein content. It has shown that a major component of the dietary specific protein leucine has extra advantages in enhancing SIRT1 to enhance fat loss and boost blood sugar regulation.

But leucine now has another role, and that's where it genuinely glows through its balanced interaction with Sirtfoods. Leucine effectively induces anabolism (building things) in our cells, especially in the muscle, which requires a great deal of energy and ensures that our energy producers (called mitochondria) have to work extra hours. It induces the need for such a Sirtfoods operation within our cells. As you may actually remember, one of the impacts of Sirtfoods is to increase the growth of more mitochondria, to increase their efficiency, and to make them blow fat as fuel. Therefore, our bodies need these to fulfill this extra demand for energy. The truth of the matter is that we see a synergistic impact when mixing Sirtfoods with dietary protein that enhances sirtuin activation and eventually allows you to lose fat to support muscle development and better safety. For this reason, the meals in the guide are built to have a reasonable protein portion.

Oily fish is an incredibly strong protein alternative to supplement Sirtfoods' action since they are high in omega-3 fatty acids alongside their nutritional value. There is no way that you may have read a lot about the health effects of oily fish and especially omega-3 fish oils. And now new evidence shows that the advantages of omega-3 fats may come from improving the functioning of our sirtuin genomes.

In recent times, questions have been presented about the harmful impact of protein-rich diets on wellbeing, without any Sirtfoods to help counter the protein; we can come to recognize why. Leucine may be a knife with two-edges. We need Sirtfoods, as we have shown, to support our cells fulfill the metabolic requirements that leucine imposes upon them. Without them, though, our mitochondria may become unstable, so elevated rates of leucine will potentially encourage obesity. Sirtfoods support to not only keep the symptoms of leucine in control but also work effectively in our favor. Assume leucine as tapping your foot on the losing weight and wellbeing accelerator, with Sirtfoods the device that guarantees that the cell fulfills the increased competition. The engine blew up, without any of the Sirtfoods.

Returning to worries about protein-rich diets' safety consequences, the missing part of the equation is Sirtfoods. Usually, most nation's diet is protein-rich, but lacks Sirtfoods to help counter it. That makes it imperative for Sirtfoods to become an essential component of how those nations feed.

Eat Early

Our ideology is superior when it comes to having a meal, preferably completing eating each day by 7 p.m. That is on two grounds. Firstly, to enjoy the Sirtfoods natural satiating power. Eating food that will leave you feeling full, happy, and energetic as you go about your day is even more effective than enduring the whole day feeling hungry enough to feed and stay full while having sleep throughout the night.

Chapter 6. What Are the Top 20 Sirtfoods and Their Benefits

The sirtfood diet comprises of a variety of different foods. The most significant benefit of a sirtfood diet is the wide variety of different food spectrums, which can be incorporated into our personalized diet plan. The sirtfood diet can also have coffee and wine, which is the most popular reason many celebrities follow this diet plan. Sirtfoods are the most common and most widely used foods in both the Western and Eastern worlds. To be very specific, sirtfoods are those which contain high levels of a chemical compound called polyphenol. This compound is not uniformly distributed in sirtfoods, but every sirtfood contains specific amounts of polyphenols. You must be thinking that why only polyphenols are being tackled here. The answer is straightforward yet very informative. Polyphenols are the compounds that are present naturally in sirtfood, and many types of research conducted on these foods have confirmed that these foods have the highest impacts when losing extra pounds of fats from the body.

However, the most famous foods in the sirtfood diet are actually twenty in number, and a significant portion of a sirtfood diet comprises these superfoods. The reason to stick this food on a more significant proportion of the sirtfood diet is the higher number of polyphenols present in these foods, which is essential to unlocking the sirtuin gene in the body. This gene is arguably the most critical gene to trigger many fat loss cycles in the human body.

The top twenty sirtfoods are:

Arugula

The critical factor is the nutritional benefits provided by this food, which is rich in very unique and rare benefits. It is an outstanding food that can be used in health promotion and anti-aging. It is also called a superfood. A vast scientific literature is dedicated to supporting this food. It contains high amounts of antioxidants, antifungal, antiviral, disinfectant, and protecting benefits. It is also essential in the reduction of cholesterol from the body and thus reduces the chances of atherosclerosis and heart attacks.

The word Rasayana is used in traditional Indian medicine, which is associated with the global benefits of arugula in the human body. Arugula is a natural coolant that can be a protective remedy during hot summers. It also has cooling effects on the liver and stomach.

100g raw arugula	
Calories	25 Cal
Fat	0.66 g
Carbs	3.65 g
Protein	2.58 g
Fiber	1.6 g

Buckwheat

Stomach acids, disturbed gut mobility and injured food canal (esophagus) cause heartburn, a condition that affects every human many times in their lives. Buckwheat prevents heartburn by improving the capacities of the stomach and colon as well as by healing the food canal. Our extensive and small intestines have bacteria called E.coli, which are friendly and help digest the food. Buckwheat is helpful to E.coli and thus improves the medium inside the large and small intestine. That helps to prevent irritable bowel syndrome and Crohn's disease, conditions that affect the colon adversely. It can effectively treat the issues related to constipation due to high concentrations of fiber.

100g buckwheat	
Calories	343 Cal
Fat	3.4 g
Carbs	71.5 g
Protein	13.25 g
Fiber	10 g

Capers

The importance of this root plant in traditional Chinese herbalism is well known. It is considered a great root to promote the self-healing capacity of the body and to maintain vital forces inside the body. Some western herbalists also used this root as the primary source of tonic, which is essential to promote natural immunity and vital capacities of the body. This root has some fantastic impacts on the neural and endocrinal systems of the body. It can be a primary herbal remedy for patients with deficient immunity or those who are treated by chemotherapy and radiotherapy.

These benefits of the herb make it an herbal remedy of choice for cancer patients all over the world. It is a primary adaptive herbal remedy in oncology. Moreover, the use of astragalus is hazard-free and safe. It has a fantastic impact on bone marrow. Thus, it can easily promote immunity by producing more potent white blood cells that can be used in the war against deadly pathogens like bacteria and viruses. It is very high in concentrations of polyphenols, which help in reducing body fats from the body.

100g capers	
Calories	33 Cal
Fat	0 g
Carbs	6.67 g
Protein	3.33 g
Fiber	3.2 g

Celery

Much like buckwheat, celery is very important for our stomach and intestine. Stomach acids, disturbed gut mobility, and an injured food canal (esophagus) cause heartburn, a condition that affects every human many times in their lives. Celery prevents heartburn by improving the capacities of the stomach and colon as well as by healing the food canal. Our large and small intestines have bacteria called E.coli, which are friendly and help digest the food. Buckwheat is helpful to E.coli and thus improves the medium inside the large and small intestine. That helps to prevent irritable bowel syndrome and Crohn's disease, conditions that affect the colon adversely. It can effectively treat the issues related to constipation due to high concentrations of fiber.

100g raw celery	
Calories	16 Cal
Fat	0.17 g
Carbs	2.97 g
Protein	0.69 g
Fiber	1.6 g

Chilies

Chilies are used in Western and Eastern foods and can be utilized to achieve higher metabolic rates because they are rich in capsicum. Capsicum is a potent fat mobilizer that can be used to break adipose tissues into much simpler precursors called fatty acid. Its action is dual. When these free fatty acids reach our blood, capsicum's action in chilies is to increase the basal metabolic rate, which is highly essential to burn these extra fatty acids in the bloodstream and thus promote a lean physique without extra fat.

100g chilies	
Calories	40 Cal
Fat	0.32 g
Carbs	9.14 g
Protein	1.94 g
Fiber	1.5 g

Cocoa

Cocoa is very important for the brain. By improving overall health and through its antioxidant properties, cocoa can reduce the chances of dementia, Parkinsonism, and much other related pathology. Fatigue is another crucial aspect to be tackled here. Mental fatigue is related to the brain's exhausting after prolonged functioning or reduced brain capacities, which can lead to general body pains and low self-esteem. By providing the nutritional supply to the brain, cocoa can help to prevent mental as well as general fatigue.

100g cocoa	
Calories	377 Cal
Fat	3 g
Carbs	71.93 g
Protein	15.49 g
Fiber	

Coffee

Coffee is the reason for the popularity of the sirtfood diet. This diet regime allows the intake of caffeine in the body to help break the adipose tissues into fatty acids. Coffee, especially caffeine anhydrous, is beneficial in the mobilization of fats. Moreover, coffee also reduces fatigue in the brain, and it helps in the promotion of mental alertness. It is the biggest cause that the sirtfood diet provides mental focus and alertness to its users, which is not provided in many other ordinary fat loss diet plans.

100g brewed coffee	
Calories	1 Cal
Fat	0.02 g
Carbs	0 g
Protein	0.12 g
Fiber	0 g

Extra-Virgin Olive Oil

Olive oil is the most used type of oil throughout the globe. Italian and French diets primarily include olive oils in the main course. Extra virgin olive oil is the lightest form of olive oil. It provides many polyunsaturated fatty acids, which are actually high-density lipids. These fatty acids are essential in reducing blood cholesterol levels and being a vital energy source in the body. Olive oil is well-researched about its benefits on the brain and cardiac health, and honestly, this attempt is not sufficient to describe the benefits of olive oil.

100g extra virgin coconut oil	
Calories	19 Cal
Fat	0.5 g
Carbs	3.71 g
Protein	0.72 g
Fiber	1.1 g

Garlic

For years garlic has been considered one of nature's wonder foods with healing and rejuvenating powers. Garlic is a powerful antioxidant, antibiotics, and antifungal often used to treat stomach ulcers. It lowers cholesterol by 10 percent and blood pressure by 5 to 7 percent, as well as blood sugar levels. The sirtuins-activating nutrients in garlic are ajoene, myricetin, and they are complemented by another key nutrient called the allicin, which gives off the characteristic aroma of garlic.

100g raw garlic	
Calories	149 Cal
Fat	05. g
Carbs	33.06 g
Protein	6.36 g
Fiber	2.1 g

Green Tea

Green tea is one of the most widely used types of tea around the world because of its health benefits. Green tea is well-researched about its benefits on the brain and cardiac health, and honestly, this writing is not sufficient to describe the benefits of olive oil. Green tea has rich historical importance in Indian ayurvedic medicine as well as in traditional western medicine. It was widely used to promote attention, focus, long-term and short term memory, and brainpower in both children and adults. It was also used as an effective tonic for the heart and vascular health. In some literature, it is also shown that it was also used in lung diseases.

100g Green tea	
Calories	1 Cal
Fat	0 g
Carbs	0.3 g
Protein	0 g
Fiber	0 g

Kale

Kale is perhaps one of the greatest, healthiest veggies that you can take advantage of—for good reason. It is by far, one of the healthiest foods that you can get, and it also happens to be a wonderful source of sirtuins. It may be a bit of an acquired taste, but over time, you can grow to love it—and you will also probably find that it is highly beneficial to your health as well. Eaten on its own, sautéed, as chips, or mixed into a salad, kale is something that you should try to consume regularly. Even better, kale is low in calories while also providing a massive amount of your nutritional value, meaning that you get the best bang for your buck, especially when you are busy restricting calories. One cup of kale, roughly 33 calories, will have over 200% of your daily value of vitamin A, nearly 700% of your vitamin K, 130% of vitamin C, and is loaded up with all sorts of other essentials as well. It also happens to be loaded up with antioxidants like beta-carotene, helping to clear out the body and offering very similar benefits to those that you can expect to see in the Sirtfood Diet.

100g raw kale	
Calories	49 Cal
Fat	0.96 g
Carbs	8.75 g
Protein	4.28 g
Fiber	3.6 g

Medjool Dates

The addition of Medjool dates at a listing of foods that spark weight loss and boosts health can come as a surprise—particularly if we inform you that Medjool dates have a staggering 66% glucose. Sugar owns no sirtuins-activating properties at all; instead, it's well-established connections for obesity, cardiovascular disease, and diabetes quite the contrary to that which we're searching to realize. But refined glucose is extremely different from sugar taken in a car supplied by the character that's balanced using sirtuins-activating polyphenols: the Medjool date. In full contrast to regular sugar Medjool dates, consumed in moderation, really don't have any real noticeable blood-sugar-raising consequences.

100g Medjool dates	
Calories	277 Cal
Fat	0.15 g
Carbs	74.97 g
Protein	1.81 g
Fiber	6.7 g

Parsley

Most people do not think of parsley as particularly healthy or even think of it when it comes to food just because it is not really needed to be consumed on its own. Rather, it is used typically in small amounts as a garnish on food. However, many people are then missing out on all of the wonderful health benefits that parsley has to offer. It is high in vitamins A, C, and K, and it is also, once again, high in antioxidants. You will see this added into the green juice as well.

100g Raw parsley	
Calories	36 Cal
Fat	0.79 g
Carbs	6.33 g
Protein	2.97 g
Fiber	3.3 g

Red Endive

As far as vegetables are concerned, chicory is a relatively new kid on the block. History says that chicory was discovered by accident with a Belgian farmer in 1830. The farmer kept chicory roots, later used as a substitute for coffee, in his basement, just to forget about them.

Upon his return, he found they had sprouted white leaves, which upon tasting that he discovered to become tender, crispy, and quite yummy. Today, the endive is increased worldwide, such as the USA, and makes its Sirtfood badge due to its remarkable content of this sirtuin activator luteolin. Besides the recognized sirtuins-activating added benefits, luteolin ingestion is getting a promising treatment approach for enhancing sociability in autistic kids. It's a crisp feel and a candy favor accompanied with a gentle and agreeable bitterness for all those new to endive.

If you are stuck on the best way best to boost endive on your diet plan, you cannot lose by incorporating its leaves into a salad, even in which its own welcome, sour favor provides the ideal snack to some zesty extra virgin olive oil-based dressing. The same as orange, onion is greatest, but the yellowish number may also be regarded as a Sirtfood. Although the red selection can sometimes be more difficult to locate, you may be certain that yellow is a totally appropriate alternate.

100g Raw endive	
Calories	17 Cal
Fat	0.2 g
Carbs	3.35 g
Protein	1.25 g
Fiber	3.1 g

Red Onions

Onions are a dietary staple as our ancient predecessors' timing, being among the first crops to be cultivated, some 5,000 decades back. With such a long history of usage and these powerful health-giving possessions, onions are admired by many civilizations that have come before us. The Egyptians maintained them in specific eminence as worship items, seeing their circle-within-a-circle arrangement as emblematic of eternal life.

Along with the Greeks thought onions fortified athletes. Ahead of the Olympic Games, athletes could consume their way through enormous quantities of onions, drinking the juice! It is an amazing testimony to the way precious early dietary wisdom may be when we believe that onions make their high twenty Sirtfood standing as they're chock-full of this sirtuins-activating chemical quercetin—that the very chemical the entire world of sports mathematics has lately begun actively exploring and promotion to enhancing sports performance. And red? Just because they have the maximum quercetin material, although conventional yellows do not stay far away, and besides, they are also a fantastic inclusion.

100g Red onions, raw	
Calories	44 Cal
Fat	0.1 g
Carbs	9.93 g
Protein	0.94 g
Fiber	2.2 g

Red Wine

Any listing of the best twenty Sirtfoods wouldn't be complete without the addition of red wine, even the most first Sirtfood. From the early 1990s, the French poet made headlines with it had been found that regardless of the French seeming to do anything wrong in regards to health (smoking, lack of practice, and ingestion of rich meals), they'd reduced death rates from cardiovascular disease compared to countries like the United States.

Doctors indicated the reason was that the copious quantities of red wine were swallowed. In 1995, Danish researchers released a function to demonstrate that low-to-moderate red wine intake reduced death rates. In contrast, comparable to alcohol, amounts of alcoholic beverages had no impact, and comparable alcohol intakes of hard liquors increased passing prices. In 2003, obviously, red wine rich material of a bevy of all sirtuins-activating nourishment was discovered, and the remainder, as they say, became background. But there is more to red wine remarkable résumé. Red wine seems to have the ability to ward off the frequent cold, using average wine drinkers using a higher than 40% decrease in its prevalence. Studies also reveal advantages for oral wellbeing and in avoidance of cavities. With average ingestion also demonstrated to boost social communication and out-of-the-box believing that after-work beverage, one of the coworkers to talk and perform endeavors seems to possess a powerful science heritage. Naturally, moderation is essential.

Only tiny quantities are required for advantage, and surplus alcohol fast undoes the great. The sweet spot is apparently sticking over US recommendations up to a single 5-ounce drink every day for women as well as 2 5-ounce beverages every day for men. To guarantee maximum sirtuins-activating bang for the dollar, wines in the New York area (particularly pinot noir, cabernet sauvignon, and merlot) possess the highest polyphenol content of the most frequently accessible wines.

1 Glass red wine	
Calories	153 Cal
Fat	0 g
Carbs	4.7 g
Protein	0.126 g
Fiber	0 g

Soy

Soy may be somewhat controversial, but it is highly healthy as well, and it will serve as a wonderful plant-based protein for your meals as you read through the recipes that will be provided to you. You will be able to introduce the plant protein to your diet, meaning that you are getting food that is lower in fats and loaded up with omega-3 and omega-6 fats, which you will need.

100g Soy	
Calories	57 Cal
Fat	0.3 g
Carbs	5.59 g
Protein	9.05 g
Fiber	0.7 g

Strawberries

Strawberries are another great source of sirtuins that also provide you with a wide range of benefits. Whether you eat them straight without preparing them, include them in a salad, toss them in yogurt, or have any other preferences regarding how you wish to consume them, there is no doubt about it—strawberries are beneficial. All you have to do is consume them. Strawberries are also high in antioxidants that are great for your heart and blood sugar. They are also quite rich in vitamin C, folate, and manganese. They are deemed a superfood for a reason, and they will leave you feeling better than ever.

100g Raw strawberries	
Calories	32 Cal
Fat	0.3 g
Carbs	7.68 g
Protein	0.67 g
Fiber	2 g

Turmeric

Turmeric pops up repeatedly in all sorts of diets, and for a good reason—it is incredibly beneficial to all sorts of people for all kinds of reasons. If you want to add a natural nutritional supplement to your life, this is it. It is highly beneficial to your brain and your body, and even better, it tastes great. Turmeric is full of curcuminoids, antioxidants that can be used to help you keep your body healthy. Turmeric is filled up with this. However, it also aids in inflammation and, therefore, would be able to help with many of the chronic diseases suffered from in the western world. Even better, it boosts these powers' ability to work by blocking free radicals and then boosting your own antioxidant enzymes to help fight against them. Essentially it is like the backup to the rest of the ingredients while also providing high levels of antioxidants. Even better, you can throw it together to make delicious curry with many of the other ingredients on this list so far.

100g Ground turmeric	
Calories	312 Cal
Fat	3.25 g
Carbs	67.14 g
Protein	9.68 g
Fiber	22.7 g

Walnuts

Walnuts are, you guessed it—rich in antioxidants. Even better, they also have the addition of omega-3 fatty acids and can help you stay fuller for longer. Whether you will eat handfuls on their own or mix them into anything else, this is a great way for you to help support your body in staying happy and healthy. These foods are often eaten plain, but you can use them in all sorts of other contexts, such as in your pasta or cereal or baking them into something. However, because they are high in fat, you will have to worry about the calorie content if you are eating them during calorie restriction. Be mindful of how many you are eating to ensure that you do not go over them when eating.

100g Walnuts	
Calories	654 Cal
Fat	65.21 g
Carbs	13.71 g
Protein	15.23 g
Fiber	6.7 g

Chapter 7. The Phases of Sirtfood Diet

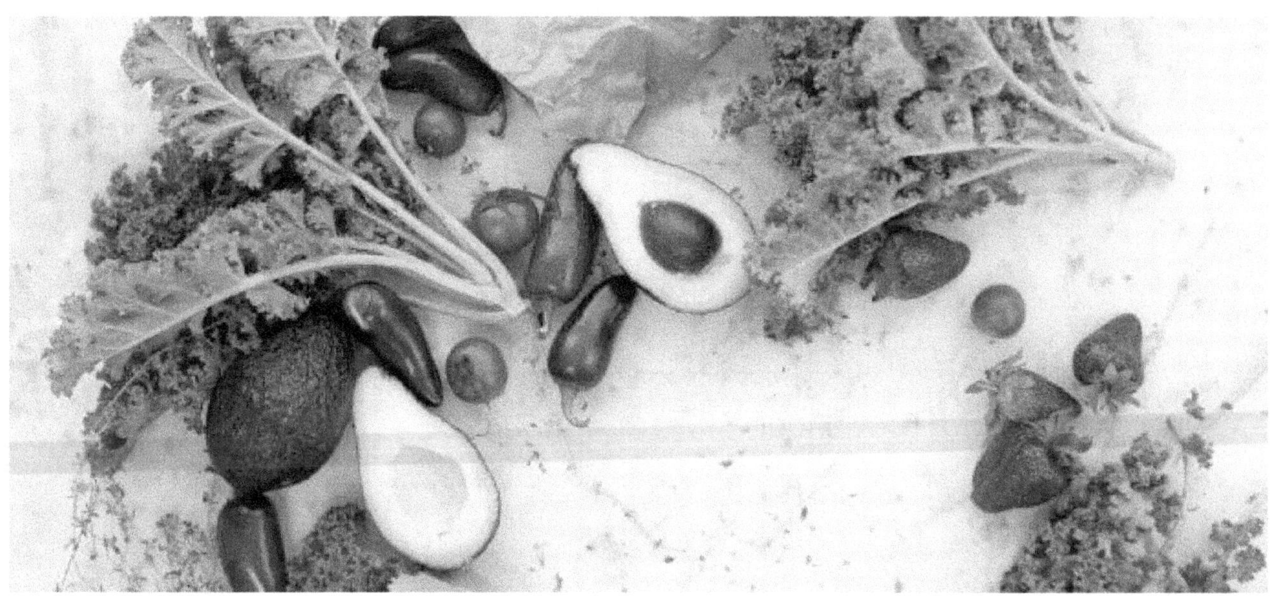

The sheer range of benefits enjoyed by people has been a surprise; all done by merely basing their diet on available and inexpensive foods that most people already enjoy consuming, and this is all that the Sirtfood Diet requires. It's about extracting the advantages of daily foods that we've all been used to consume, but in the right proportions and formulations to give us the body structure and health we need.

Everybody desires something very desperately, and that will fundamentally change our lives.

It doesn't require you to execute extreme calorie restrictions, nor does it require grueling exercise regimens (although staying consistently active is a good thing, of course). And just a juicer is the only piece of equipment you'll require.

How to follow the Sirtfood Diet

Most sirtfoods and ingredients are easy to find.

A big part of the diet is green tea, which you'll have to make between one and three times a day. A juicer (a blender won't work) and a kitchen scale will be needed, as the ingredients are listed by weight.

Phase 1: Slimming

Welcome to Sirtfood Diet, phase 1. This is the process of hyper-success, where you will take a huge step towards achieving a slimmer, leaner body. Follow our simple step-by-step instructions and use the tasty recipes you'll get. We do have a meat-free option in addition to our regular seven-day program, which is ideal for vegetarians and vegans alike. Feel free to go ahead with whatever you want.

What to Expect

You'll reap the full benefits of our clinically proven method of losing 7 pounds in seven days during Phase 1. But note that involves adding weight, so don't hang up simply on the numbers on the scales. Nor should you get used to measuring yourself every day. Besides, in the last few days of Phase 1, we always see the scales rising due to muscle growth, while waistlines tend to shrink. Therefore, we want you to look at the dimensions but not be controlled by them. Check out how you feel inside the mirror, if your clothing matches, or whether you need to push a knot on your belt. These are all perfect measures of the greater changes in body composition.

Be mindful of other improvements, too, such as well-being, energy levels, and how clean the skin appears. At the local pharmacy, you can get tests of your general cardiovascular and metabolic well-being to see improvements in factors like blood pressure, blood sugar levels, and blood fats like cholesterol and triglycerides. Remember, weight loss aside, introducing Sirtfoods into your diet is a huge step in making your cells fitter and more disease resistant, setting you up for an exceptional healthy lifetime.

How to Follow Phase 1

To make Step 1 sailing as simple as possible, we will lead you one day at a time through the full seven-day schedule, including the Sirtfood Green Juice lowdown and quick to follow tasty recipes every step of the way.

Phase 1 of the Sirtfood Diet is built on two specific stages:

Days one to three are the highest demanding, and during this time, you can consume up to a limit of 1,000 calories per day, consisting of:

- Three times Sirtfood green juices

- One-time vital meal

Days four to seven will see your food consumption increase to a limit of 1,500 calories per day, consisting of the following:

- Two times Sirtfood green juices

- Two times vital meals

There are very few rules by which to obey the diet. Ultimately, for sustained progress, it's about incorporating it into the lifestyle and around daily life.

What to Drink

As well as the required daily servings of green juices, other beverages can be easily drunk in Step 1. Those should be non-calorie foods, ideally straight coke, black coffee, and green tea. If your usual tastes are for black or herbal teas, do not hesitate to add these too. Apple juices and soft drinks are left behind. Instead, consider adding a few sliced strawberries to still or sparkling water to make your Sirtfood-infused health cocktail if you want to spice things up.

Hold it for a few hours in the fridge, and you can have a surprisingly cooling alternative to soft drinks and juices. One thing you ought to be mindful of is that we don't suggest abrupt major improvements to your daily coffee use. Caffeine withdrawal symptoms may make you feel lousy for a few days; likewise, large increases may be unpleasant for those especially sensitive to caffeine effects. Since some researchers have found that adding milk will reduce the absorption of beneficial nutrients that activate sirtuin, we also recommend drinking coffee black without adding milk. The same has been found for green tea, although adding some lemon juice increases its nutrient absorption to activate sirtuin.

Remember that this is the period of hyper-success, and while you can be comforted by the fact that it is just for a week, you need to be a bit more careful. We have alcohol for this week, in the form of red wine but only as a cooking ingredient.

The Sirtfood Green Juice

The green juice is an integral component of the Sirtfood Diet's Step 1 program. All the fixings are prevailing Sirtfoods, and in every liquid, you get a strong cocktail of expected compounds like apigenin, kaempferol, luteolin, quercetin, and EGCG that work together to switch on your sirtuin genes and encourage fat damage. To that, we have added lemon, as it has been shown that its natural acidity prevents, stabilizes and improves the absorption of the sirtuins-activating nutrients. We added a touch of apple and ginger to taste too. But all of these are available. Indeed, many people notice that they take the apple out entirely until they become used to the flavor of the fruit.

Days one to three of Phase 1: combined only to the first two juices of the day.

Days four to seven of Phase 1: combined to both juices.

Note that while we weighted all the amounts exactly as described in our pilot experiment, our experience is that a handful of measures perform exceptionally well. Besides, they are better tailoring the number of nutrients to the body type of a person. Bigger people tend to have larger paws, and therefore, get a proportionally higher volume of Sirtfood nutrients to suit their body size and vice versa.

Phase 2: Maintenance

Having witnessed these sometimes-incredible transformations ourselves, we know how often you're going to want to see much greater outcomes, not just retain all the advantages. Sirtfoods are, after all, built to eat for life. The problem is how you adapt what you did in Step 1 into your normal dietary routine. That's exactly what prompted us to create a 14-day follow-up maintenance plan designed to help you transition from Phase 1 to your more normal nutritional routine, thereby maintaining and extending the benefits of the Diet Sirtfood.

What to Expect

You will consolidate your weight loss results during Phase 2 and continue to lose weight steadily. Also, the one surprising point we've seen with the Sirtfood Diet is that much or all of the weight people lose is from fat, and that many even add some muscle in. We would like to warn you again not to measure your success solely based on the numbers. Look in the mirror to see how you feel leaner and more toned, see how well your suits match, and soak up the compliments you'll get from everyone.

How to Follow Phase 2

All you need to do is replicate the Seven Day Schedule twice to complete Step 2's fourteen days.

Once again, there are no particular guides for when you have to take these. Be soft and fit them around your day.

Portion Sizes

During Step 2, our attention is not on calorie counting. For the average person, this is not a practical or successful approach over the long term. Instead, we concentrate on healthy servings, very well-balanced meals, and most notably, stocking up on Sirtfoods so that you can start to benefit from their fat-burning and health-promoting effects.

We've also built the meals in the plan to make them satiate, helping you feel full for longer. That, coupled with Sirtfoods' natural appetite-regulating powers, means you're not going to spend the next 14 days feeling thirsty, but instead happily relaxed, well-fed, and highly well-nourished. Just like in Phase 1, remember to listen and be guided by your appetite. When you prepare meals according to our guidelines and find that you are easily full before you finish a meal, then stop eating perfectly!

What to Drink

Throughout Step 2, you'll have to have one green juice daily. This is to keep you top with high Sirtfoods levels. Much as in Phase 1, you can easily absorb other fluids in Phase 2. Our favorite drinks include remaining plain water, homemade flavored water, coffee, and green tea. If black or white tea is your preference, feel free to indulge. The same goes for herbal teas. The great thing is that during Step 2, you will enjoy the occasional bottle of red wine. Due to its content of sirtuins-activating polyphenols, particularly resveratrol and piceatannol, red wine is a sirtfood, which makes it by far the best choice of alcoholic beverage. But, with alcohol itself causing harmful effects on our fat cells, restraint is always safest, so we suggest restricting the drink to one glass of red wine with a meal for two to three days a week during Step 2.

Returning to Three Meals

Having a healthy breakfast sets us ready for the day, raising our levels of vitality and focus. Eating earlier keeps our blood sugar and fat levels in check, in terms of our metabolism. A variety of studies point out that breakfast is a positive idea, usually finding that people who eat breakfast are often less likely to be overweight.

The explanation for this is because our body clocks inside. Our bodies ask us to feed early in expectation of when we will be busiest and need food. Yet, as many as a third of us will miss breakfasts on every given day. It's a typical example of our crazy everyday life and the impression that there's just not enough time to eat properly. But as you will see, nothing could be further from the truth with the nifty breakfasts we have laid out for you. If it's the Sirtfood smoothie that can be drunk on the go, the premade Sirt muesli, or the fast and simple Sirtfood scrambled eggs/tofu, having those extra few minutes in the morning will yield rewards not only for your day but also for your weight and well-being over the longer term.

What About Snacking?

Snacks have been branded as the devil incarnate. "To lose weight, you have to give up snacks," how many times have you heard it?

It's not true; if you have had a busy day and your rushing between work, home, and getting around with kids, it's perfectly normal to need something to tide you over between meals. You can enjoy some guilt-free treats made entirely out of Sirtfoods!

"Sirtifying" Your Meals

The thinking goes, if it's just for three weeks, I can eat anything… But this shouldn't be the case with the Sirtfood diet. You shouldn't constantly worry about food restrictions, just take a look at the recipe, and you will realize that they are clever, tasty twists on classics. So, they will be easy to incorporate into your life and the life of those around you, be it children or fussy hosts. Examples include the delicious Sirtfood smoothie for the perfect on-the-go breakfast, and the simple switch from wheat to buckwheat for adding extra taste and zip to what seemed the guilty-pleasure of pasta.

Meanwhile, iconic, beloved dishes such as chili con carne and curry don't even need much change, with the traditional recipes offering Sirtfood goodness. And who said fast-food meant bad food? Find the authentic, vibrant flavors of a pizza and remove the guilt by making it yourself. There's no need to say farewell to indulgence either, as proven by our pancakes laden with berries and dark chocolate sauce. It's not even dessert, it's breakfast, and it's great for you. Simple changes: you continue to eat the foods you love while driving a healthy weight and well-being. And that is the dietary revolution that is Sirtfoods.

Don't Stick to Just the Top 20 Sirtfoods

The top 20 sirtfoods are great sources of SIRT-activating ingredients, but that doesn't mean that you should only eat those for the rest of your life. There are other ingredients that are healthy and have analogue SIRT-activating functions. Goggins and Mattens have only picked out the best of the best. But feel free to expand your diet. Actually you are encouraged to do it to achieve a more balanced lifestyle and continued wellbeing.

How About Proteins?

Proteins are a staple of the Sirtfood diet, as you will see in the recipes. You can consume eggs, dairy, poultry, and red meat. Just stay away from processed meat, or at least reduce their consumption significantly. Vegans should be mindful of integrating iodine, calcium, and vitamin B12, but that is true for any diet.

Tips for Cooking with Sirtfoods

When trying to cook with the sirtfoods, most of the ingredients you should be familiar with already. However, there are a few which will be new.

Matcha is green tea, but in a powdered form. You're unlikely to be able to buy it from the shelves of your local supermarket, but it will be available from health specialist stores or online retailers. Matcha is generally produced in China and Japan, where it is a traditional beverage, so you should expect to order from overseas.

It is better if you can buy Matcha from Japan, as Matcha from China may have forms of pollution and impurities due to the environment. Matcha green tea is used in Zen ceremonies in Japan, and it is even better for you than regular green tea. The unique nature of Matcha green tea originates from how it is grown. Matcha is grown almost entirely in dark shadowy environments, while green tea is usually grown in bright sunshine.

Matcha is also ground into a powder using a mill, rather than being cut into small leaves and added as an infusion.

Lovage is another ingredient you probably have never heard of. Lovage is an herb, but one that hasn't been used by our culinary society for over 100 years. It can be bought, but it is more practical to grow your own. Lovage plants are low maintenance—you should be able to plant the seeds in a regular pot, put it on the windowsill in your house, water it once a day, and see growth in a few weeks. Lovage seeds will be available from most garden centers (or you can buy an already thriving plant).

Additionally, you may or may not have heard of buckwheat. Buckwheat is a grain that is high in protein, carbohydrates, and sirtuin. However, other foods made from buckwheat, such as buckwheat pasta or soba noodles, will need to either be bought online or sourced from a specialist store.

Owing to this, if you are not well-acquainted with spicy foods, you should reduce the amount you add to your recipes, to begin with. Try half the recommended value, ensuring you de-seed the chili as the seeds themselves are rather spicy.

Miso is a type of soya-bean paste, which is used for flavoring in eastern dishes. Miso comes in multiple flavors, with the lighter colored variants being sweeter than the darker colors. You can experiment with what flavor suits you best. In a similar vein, the miso's potency varies between the different colors (white, yellow, red & brown), so you might want to lower or increase the amount of miso you use to get the taste just right.

Buckwheat should be washed before it is cooked by placing it in a sieve and rinsing it with water. Flat-leaf parsley is preferable to curly leaf, but the latter is acceptable if you cannot source the former.

Finally, feel free to season and add salt and pepper as necessary, although the recipes are intended to be tasty without additional flavoring.

Chapter 8. Questions and Answers

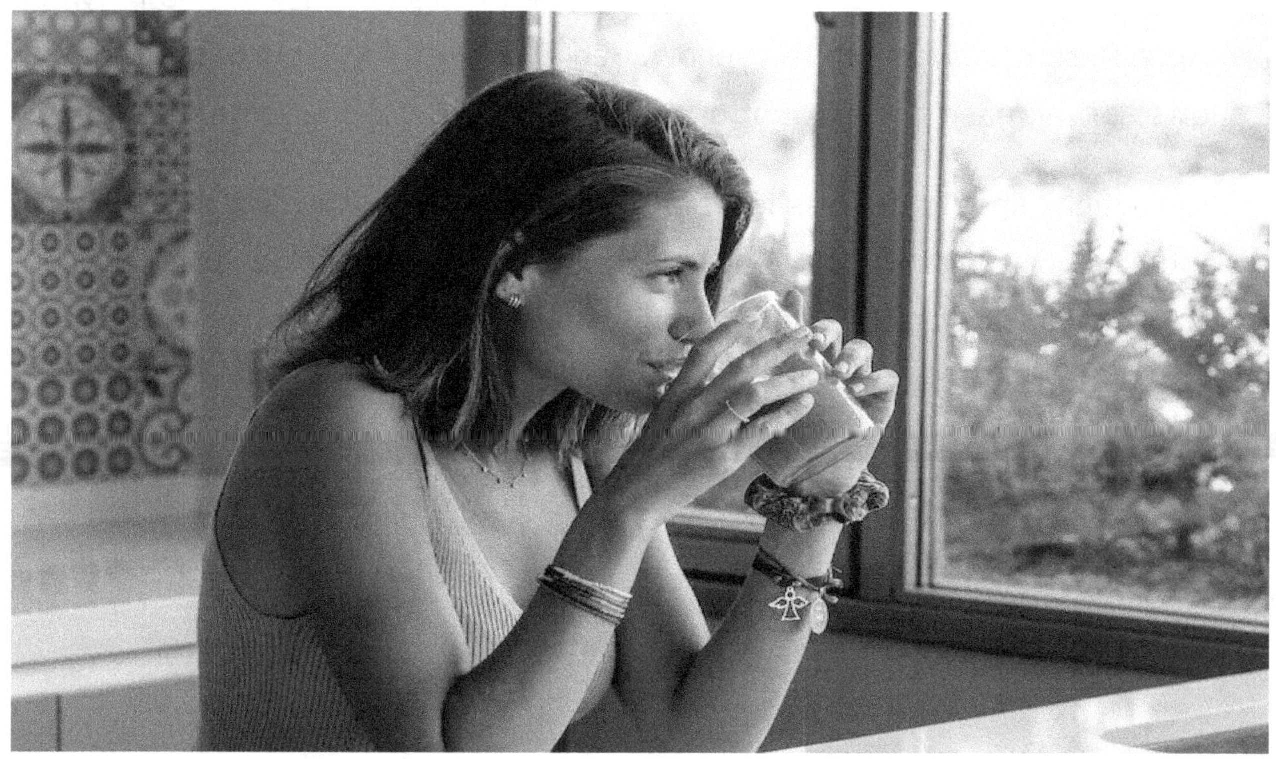

Would It Be Advisable for Me to Exercise During Stage 1?

Ordinary exercise is perhaps the best thing you can accomplish for your wellbeing, and doing some direct exercise will improve the weight-loss and medical advantages of Stage 1 of the diet. When in doubt, we urge you to proceed with your typical degree of activity and physical movement through the initial seven days of the Sirtfood Diet. Be that as it may, we recommend remaining inside your typical safe place, since delayed or excessively exceptional exercise may basically put a lot of weight on the body for this period. Tune in to your body. There's no compelling reason to push you to accomplish more exercise during Stage 1; let the Sirtfoods perform the difficult work.

I'm Now Thin—Would I Be Able to In Any Case Follow the Diet?

We don't suggest Stage 1 of the Sirtfood Diet for any underweight individual. A decent method to see whether you are underweight is to compute your weight record or BMI. For whatever length of time that you know your tallness and weight, you can without much of a stretch, decide this by utilizing one of the various BMI number crunchers on the web. In the event that your BMI is 18.5 or less, we don't suggest that you leave on Stage 1 of the diet. If your BMI is somewhere in the range of 18.5 and 20, we will look at present urge alert, since following the diet may imply that your BMI falls underneath 18.5.

Even the Sirtfood Diet Measures Success Just Concerning Weight Loss

Weight is a determinant of health. However, it is perhaps not the just person. To quantify somebody's health success on if or not they lose x pounds in x timeframe dismisses the rest of the advantages of food. Food is active, which lets you complete such things as showering, breathing, and exercising. Additionally, it has nutrients that could promote several physiological functions and can be many times a happy experience rooted in the convention. For overall wellness, there is much more to give attention to than appearance, and quantifying success just concerning losing weight is comprehensive.

It's Restrictive, and That May Harm Your Relationship

This diet highlights the ingestion of 1000 to 1,500 calories every day, which will be far below a lot of men and women need. If we severely restrict our food ingestion, our instinctive reaction will be to overeat. Your own body is sensible, and it believes that the shortage of sustenance within an attack. For that reason, we are inclined to overcompensate, which explains precisely why we can connect with becoming "hangry" and thus over-indulging when we're finally allowed to eat. Practicing careful and intuitive eating is a much more sustainable path than limiting meals.

Is Sirtfood Diet Science-Based?

Even though there's some contentious research in regard to the advantages of Sirtuins, there is little to no research in regards to the particular Sirtfood dietary plan. In any case, we have any tips in place, which were thoroughly researched and analyzed for many years. If you should be lost about which "healthy food" is, then this can be a higher place to get started.

It is beautiful if you'd like to add some Sirtfoods in an eating program. After all, foods such as green tea extract, tea, chocolate brown, and kale all have an area within a nutritious eating pattern! But staying with a schedule with such strict pass-or-fail conditions is unrealistic and may be inadequate for your relationship with food. By incorporating a diet plan that is full of numbers and eating mindfully, you are going to be in a position to set a long-term and sustainable romance with food. Cheers to this!

Five Truth Practically Everybody Makes Sirtfood Diet

Eating Foods That You Cannot Actually Like

In case you believe you are going to turn into a fan of Brussels sprouts as its January second and you've not eaten anything in the previous three months weeks, you are setting yourself up to fail. One explanation of why diet does not work is because they induce people to eat things that they don't like. "If the carrot smoothie isn't exercising for you, take to sautéed lettuce, celery, tofu chips, or even better, ditch the carrot and attempt lettuce, collard greens, Swiss chard, or still another vegetable. The following secret to eating healthy without quitting life would be really to test out spices." Do not forget to take to various seasonings or manners of cooking. By way of instance, get a Cajun spice combination or five-spice and scatter it together with one's poultry or veggies.

Expecting Immediate Results

The observing you did on Christmas isn't going to become reversed following weekly—or possibly (i.e., Healthy eating). "The most straightforward way to fall short of one's resolution or goal is to help it become unattainable." Lead nourishment specialist at Seattle Sutton's healthy eating. For example, hoping to avoid eating your favorite take-out food or planning to lose 10 pounds, within one month may backfire. That is not because allowing the foods that you like results in finally bingeing to them once you cannot tolerate the craving, and seeking to reduce a lot of weight too fast will undoubtedly cause disappointment and also a dip bag of Doritos.

The key would be to put smaller goals that build-up to an objective, he states. This means that you may attempt to prevent this take out joint more frequently than you can today or wish to lose a couple of pounds weekly—and soon you finally reach your target," she states.

Maybe Not Getting Meals in Front of Time

One of the reasons why people overeat around Christmas is there is a large amount of food outside. It is easy to catch. Whenever the observing is finished, make it simple to choose healthful options by organizing healthy food beforehand. Like that, it is possible to arrive at it when you are hungry, rather than earning a game-time decision when you are mesmerized. Meal preparation is critical to eating a balanced diet program. Cut vegetables up and also make additional portions of dinner to the week beforehand. In this manner, it is possible to collect dinner for a busy week very quickly.

Now you won't think some of the strangest things a few individuals did to eliminate weight:

Maybe Not Assessing Labels at the Supermarket

Being a little more particular regarding the foods that you buy at the store will be able to assist you in getting right back on the right track after ingestion that which without any difficulty. Examine the food labels to the ingredients you have to produce a more informed decision regarding whether it belongs in what you eat plan. Chen says it mainly crucial to pay careful attention to serving sizes. "A jar of juice might comprise two portions," she states. This means it includes twice the calories and sugar just as what's recorded on the tag, and as you are not likely in the habit of just drinking half a juice, then which will prevent you from losing weight. Other critical elements to consider will be the total amount of protein and fiber in meals. Take 2 g of fiber and 20 g of protein into every meal to remain full and fulfilled.

Maybe Not Acquiring a Backup Policy for Seconds Weakness

Putting a strategy set up to modify your daily diet is fantastic. However, you've also must policy for roadblocks. Simply take stress eating throughout a mainly annoying afternoon. Once you learn, you are enticed to make yourself feel a lot better with the assistance of ice cream, then look for a backup program. Maybe you opt to find yourself a 20-minute massage at a nail salon or blow some steam off from the particular candlelight yoga class. "Both are welcome adjustments to a healthier new way of life, and you'll feel far better in the long term."

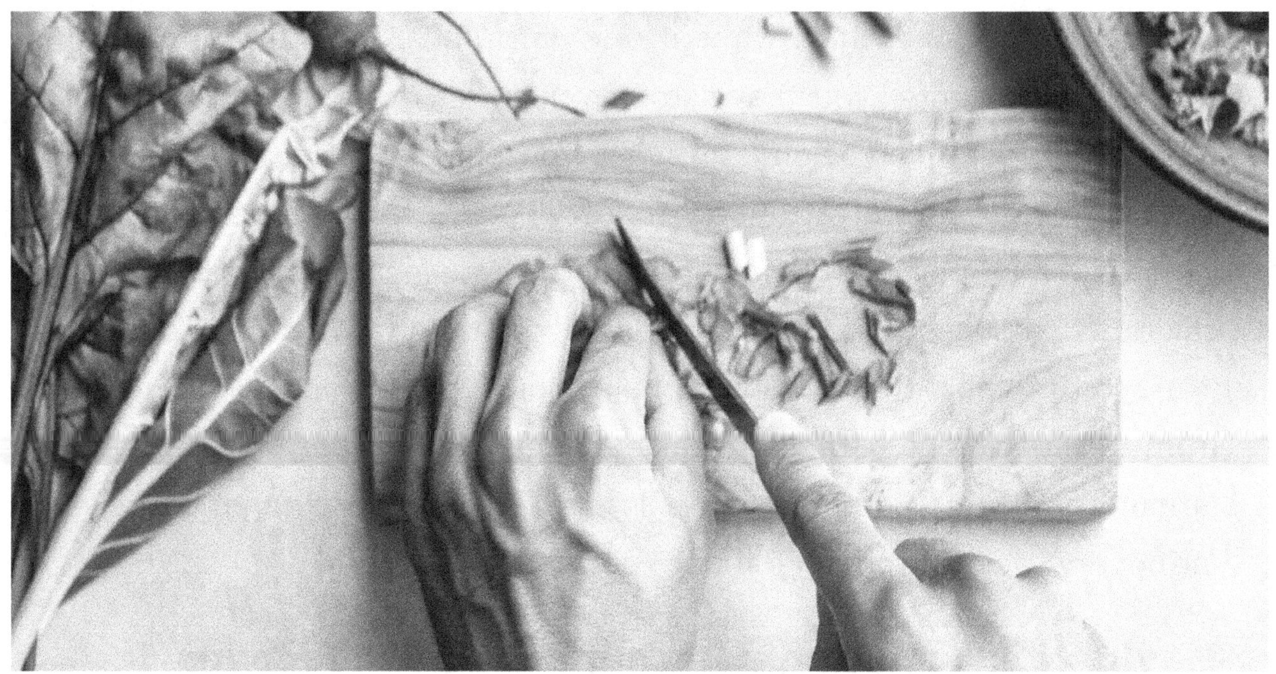

I'm Corpulent—Is the Sirtfood Diet Directly for Me?

Indeed! Try not to be put off by the way that lone a little minority of the members who set out on our pilot study were corpulent. This is on the grounds that the pilot study was done in a wellbeing and wellness club where individuals are commonly fitter and more wellbeing cognizant. Rather, be prodded on by the way that the rare sorts of people who were corpulent had stunningly better outcomes than our healthy-weight members. These outcomes have been reproduced by many great individuals who have attempted the diet in reality. In view of the investigation into sirtuin actuation, you ought to likewise remain to harvest the best changes in your prosperity. Being corpulent builds the danger of various incessant medical issues, yet these are the very sicknesses that Sirtfoods help to ensure against.

I've arrived at My Objective Weight and Would Prefer Not to Lose Any More—Do I Quit Eating Sirtfoods?

In the first place, congrats on your weight-loss accomplishment! You've had incredible achievement with Sirtfoods; however, it doesn't end now. While we don't suggest further calorie limitation, your diet should, in any case, give sufficient Sirtfoods. A significant number of our customers are currently at their optimal body structure; however, keeping on eating Sirtfood-rich diets. The incredible thing about Sirtfoods is that they are a lifestyle. The most ideal approach is to consider them concerning weight the board is that they help carry the body to the weight and synthesis it was intended to be. From here, they work to keep up and keep you looking and feeling incredible.

I've Completed Stage 2—Do I Quit Drinking the Morning Sirtfood Green Squeeze Now?

The green juice is our preferred method to get an awesome hit of Sirtfoods to begin the day, so we embrace its drawn-out utilization. Our Sirtfood green juice was deliberately intended to incorporate fixings that give a full range of sirtuins-actuating supplements in powerful fat-consuming and prosperity boosting dosages. In any case, we are totally supportive of assortment, and keeping in mind that we do suggest you proceed with a morning juice, we completely bolster anybody hoping to try different things with various Sirtfood juice creations.

I Take Drug—Is It Alright to Follow the Diet?

The Sirtfood Diet is appropriate for a great many people, but since of its ground-breaking consequences for fat consuming and wellbeing, it can change certain malady forms and the activities of prescription recommended by your primary care physician. In like manner, certain drugs are not reasonable in a fasting state. During the preliminary of the Sirtfood Diet, we surveyed the appropriateness of every individual before the person in question left on a diet, particularly the individuals who were taking prescription.

Would I Be Able to Follow the Diet In Case I'm Pregnant?

We don't suggest leaving on the Sirtfood Diet on the off chance that you are attempting to consider or in the event that you are pregnant or breastfeeding. It is an incredible weight-loss diet, which makes it unacceptable. In any case, don't be put off eating a lot of Sirtfoods, since these are particularly healthy nourishments to incorporate as a component of a decent and differed diet for pregnancy. You will need to stay away from red wine, because of its liquor substance, and cutoff stimulated things, for example, espresso, green tea, and cocoa so as not to surpass 200 milligrams for each day of caffeine during pregnancy (one cup of moment espresso ordinarily contains around 100 milligrams of caffeine).

Are Sirtfoods Appropriate for Youngsters?

The Sirtfood Diet is an amazing weight-loss diet and not intended for youngsters. In any case, that doesn't imply that youngsters should pass up the phenomenal medical advantages offered by incorporating more Sirtfoods in their general diet. A greater part of Sirtfoods speak to incredibly healthy nourishments for youngsters and assist them with accomplishing adjusted and nutritious diets. A large number of the plans intended for Stage 2 of the diet were made in light of families, including youngsters' taste buds. Any semblance of the Sirtfood pizza, the bean stew with meat, and the Sirtfood nibbles are flawless kid agreeable nourishments with a nutritional worth better than common food contributions for kids.

Will I Get a Migraine or Feel Tired During Stage 1?

Stage 1 of the Sirtfood Diet gives incredible normally happening food mixes in sums that the vast majority would not get in their ordinary diet, and certain individuals can respond as they adjust to this sensational nutritional change. This can incorporate manifestations, for example, a gentle migraine or tiredness, despite the fact that we would say these impacts are minor and brief.

Obviously, if side effects are serious or give you purpose behind concern, we suggest you look for brief clinical counsel.

Would It Be a Good Idea for Me to Take Enhancements?

Except if explicitly endorsed for you by your primary care physician or other social insurance proficient, we don't suggest aimless utilization of nutritional enhancements. You will ingest a huge and synergistic cluster of characteristic plant mixes from Sirtfoods, and it is these that will benefit you. You can't repeat these advantages with nutritional enhancements and, truth be told, some nutritional enhancements, for example, cell reinforcements, particularly whenever taken at high portions, may really meddle with the helpful impacts of Sirtfoods, which is the exact opposite thing you need.

How Regularly Would I Be Able to Rehash Stages 1 and 2?

Stage 1 can be rehashed on the off chance that you sense that you need a weight-loss or wellbeing help. To guarantee that there are no drawn-out negative impacts to your digestion from calorie limitation, you should hold up, in any event, a month prior to rehashing. Be that as it may, we really locate that the vast majority need to rehash it no more regularly than once like clockwork probably and keep on getting astounding outcomes. Rather, if you find that you have deviated from the course, need a little adjustment or need more strength from Sirtfood, we suggest that you repeat a few days or all days in the Stage 2 area as regularly as you wish. All things considered, Stage 2 is tied in with setting up a lifelong method of eating.

Does the Sirtfood Diet Give Enough Fiber?

Numerous Sirtfoods are normally rich in fiber. Onions, endive, and pecans are striking sources, with buckwheat and Medjool dates truly sticking out, implying that a Sirtfood-rich diet doesn't miss the mark in the fiber office. In any event, during Stage 1, when food utilization is diminished, the greater part of us will at present be devouring a fiber amount we are utilized to, particularly on the off chance that we pick the plans that contain buckwheat, beans, and lentils from the menu choices.

I've Found Out about Super Nourishments— Would It Be Advisable for Me to Incorporate These in My Diet As Well?

The main thing you have to think about the term superfood is that it's anything, but a logical term at everything except a showcasing motto. You don't have to worry about supposed super nourishments on the grounds that the Sirtfood Diet unites the most advantageous food sources on earth into a progressive better approach for eating. Similarly, as it is wrong to depend on taking a simple nutrient pill to make us healthy, it is also wrong to depend on a solitary superfood to do the same. It is the entire diet, comprised of a wide range of Sirtfoods and their huge range of normal mixes, acting in cooperative energy that is the genuine mystery to accomplishing weight loss and lifelong wellbeing.

Do I Need to Do Stage 1 For Seven Days—Would I Be Able to Do Less?

There's nothing otherworldly about Stage 1 being seven days. It is basically what we chose for our preliminary. We picked that since it was long enough to get amazing outcomes; however, not all that long that it got difficult. It likewise fits perfectly into individuals' lives. Seven days is what was tried and what is demonstrated to be compelling. In any case, if for reasons unknown you find that you have to stop it by a day or two, do as such by finishing up to the finish of Day 5 or Day 6. Try not to stress; you will find at present harvest a lot of the advantages.

Would I Be Able to Eat Anything I Desire Once I Eat a Lot of Sirtfoods and Still Get Results?

One of the key reasons the Sirtfood Diet works so well long haul is that it advances great food as opposed to deriding awful food. Diets of rejection basically don't work long haul. The facts confirm that handled nourishments that are high in sugars and fats lessen sirtuins movement in the body. In this manner, high utilization will diminish the advantages of Sirtfoods. In any case, on the off chance that you maintain your emphasis on expending a diet rich in Sirtfoods, in our experience you will find that you are charmingly fulfilled and will have less want for those prepared nourishments and wind up devouring far less garbage than the normal individual accordingly.

Would I Be Able to Eat the Same Number of Sirtfoods, Even the Unhealthy Ones, as I Like and Still Get Thinner?

Truly! Keep in mind, calories and the drive to tally them is present-day "headway." As for the way of life and the incalculable ages that have benefited from Sirtfoods, such an idea did not exist, and basically, there was no need. Individuals ate as they felt like it, and remained thin and liberated from infection. Given Sirtfoods' consequences for managing digestion and hunger, you just don't have to stress over eating an excessive number of them.

While this isn't a solicitation to everything you-can-eat challenge, don't hesitate to eat as much Sirtfood as you like to fulfill your regular hunger. Our one special case is Medjool dates.

Conclusion

Thank you for making it to the end. It is time people should eventually realize that they need not starve themselves before they can lose weight. All they need is to diet in sirtfoods, which has recently been proven to be a very effective way of losing weight and shedding fat while gaining muscle at the same time. As already explained in the book, sirtfood diets have quite several advantages over all other menus. It is imperative to get ourselves informed that sirtfoods are full of healthy food, but it is not an entirely healthy eating pattern. Although the sirtfood diet is undisputedly one of the best diets in the world right now, it is very costly, so the majority of the world's population cannot afford it.

For this reason, most people who use this diet are people who can afford to eat right and healthy food. Sirtfoods are easy to make—they do not require any particular skill before you prepare them. As we can see, many celebrities have undergone this diet, showing that the diet does not require much time.

We neither need to starve ourselves nor need to wage war against food before we get the excellent body we crave for. We need to ask questions like, "Why do people feel that they need to eat, why do they feel like they will die if they do not eat at least three times a day, why do they feel they are performing some kind of sacrifice if anytime they don't eat?." We also do not need to question the importance of food because food is undisputedly essential. We have to strictly adhere to the laid down instructions and suggestions made by the renowned nutritionist that made sirtfood diet known to the world.

We do not need to become extremists, all in the name of losing weight. Too much exercise, just like any other thing in the universe, is hazardous

to our health. It can cause hormonal disorder, which might ever obesity (if testosterone is affected). It can lead to fatigue when the stress hormone is altered; it can easily strain one's body injured; it can also lead to overeating. In this situation, the body burn muscle instead of fat.

All this being said, we can easily finalize that sirtfoods diet is the b in the universe now, it is easy and natural to do, it does not extreme exercise, and it does not require starvation of the person these are just one of the reasons we have to admit that no other d be compared to the sirtfood diet in recent years. The 700+ provided you will help you get on your feet. Whether you choose the plan exactly how I designed, customize it, or create your ow scratch, you will find that by having a plan and guide to follow healthier, losing weight and boosting your health can be easier than I hope you have learned something!